Repor
RISK

A Journalist's Handbook on Environmental Risk Assessment

by
Michael A Kamrin
Dolores J. Katz
Martha L. Walter

Produced by
Foundation for American Communications and
National Sea Grant College Program

CONTENTS

INTRODUCTION

Qualitative risk assessment has its roots in the beginning of human history. For example, people observed that human exposure to particular plants, such as hemlock, led to adverse health effects. In addition, they noted that some beneficial materials, such as wine, had adverse effects when taken in excess. As a result, they recognized both qualitatively and quantitatively that some products of the environment posed risks. In the main, the effects they noted were those that occurred almost immediately. Long-term effects were difficult to discern, especially when life spans were short and other health problems, particularly infectious diseases, were more prevalent.

Although the situation changed somewhat over the centuries, it was not until the present century that humans learned how to control infectious diseases. As a result, people have been living longer and have experienced an increased incidence of chronic health problems. Coincidentally, modern society has learned to synthesize a large variety of chemicals and to extract and manipulate naturally occurring chemicals. Some of the resulting chemical exposures have contributed to an increase of chronic diseases, especially cancer.

To protect the public from long-term adverse health effects from chemical exposures, a large number of environmental and occupational statutes have been enacted since 1970. Most of these laws and associated rules require that the risk from chemicals be assessed, whether the chemicals are in the workplace, the ambient air, water, soil, or food supply. The results of the risk assessments are used to set limits on environmental or workplace levels of these chemicals.

As a result of the regulatory needs for consistent rules, a number of risk assessment approaches were codified in policy years ago. Unfortunately, they reflect the state of science as it was decades ago and do not incorporate current understanding of the different ways chemicals cause toxicity. Thus, there is an increasing gap between the scientist's best judgment about the risk of chemicals and the official risk assessment numbers that are most commonly released to the press and public by government agencies.

The purpose of this primer is to give the reporter an understanding of how risk assessment is currently practiced and publicized. It is intended to enable the journalist to sort through the numbers and scientific terminology to detect whether they are getting the whole story and to identify the strengths and weaknesses of a study. The ultimate goal is to improve public understanding and decision-making regarding environmental risks.

In this handbook, risk assessment refers to the process of estimating the type and magnitude of risk to human health posed by exposure to chemical substances. The handbook does not cover chemical risks to wildlife or other types of risk. Many of the principles of risk assessment described, however, also apply to measuring other forms of risk.

This handbook distills the basics of risk assessment. It is designed to give the reader an overview of the process, what it can achieve, its limitations, and problems to watch for. It will not make the reader an expert on risk assessment, but it should provide an elementary knowledge of basic concepts and enable reporters to approach risk stories with more confidence and knowledge.

HOW TO USE THIS HANDBOOK

User's Guide

This book is designed so that the reader can easily find information on a particular topic. However, you are encouraged to read through the entire book, because the concepts build one upon another to some extent. It is also useful to leaf through the book reading the sidebars on each page. These encapsulate the information on each page, and you can then choose pages to read in more detail. *Figure 1*, on page 14, provides a quick overview of the major steps in the science of risk assessment.

There are several ways to use *Reporting on Risk* as a handbook. One is to turn to the *Key Questions* at the beginning of each chapter. These are crucial points you can cover, either when interviewing someone or when reading or hearing a report on risk. The key questions will help you determine how valid a study is.

If a term used by toxicologists or epidemiologists comes to your attention, use the *Glossary* for a quick definition of the term, and to find the text pages where the term is discussed more completely. An *Index* includes additional terms, and lists text pages where these are discussed.

In the text, words defined in the *Glossary* are introduced in *italics*. When a technical word is introduced in the text, but not described thoroughly until a later page, the word is either defined at the bottom of that page or cross-referenced.

If you would like more information, turn to Appendix 2, *Information Resources and Contacts*, for 800 numbers of a variety of organizations that can help you. The *Recommended Reading* list will lead you to publications that delve into particular areas of interest.

Appendix 1, *Concentration Analogies*, will help you visualize terms like parts per million.

ACKNOWLEDGMENTS

This handbook is the result of the dedicated efforts of many people. Many individuals with technical expertise carefully reviewed draft manuscripts and provided valuable comments and insights. These were: Anne Sweeney, Department of Human Medicine, MSU; Marie Swanson, Cancer Center, MSU; Patricia Peyser, Department of Epidemiology, UM; Christine Johnson, Division of Biostatistical Research, Henry Ford Hospital, Detroit; Dorothy Patton, Risk Assessment Forum, U.S. EPA; Nigel Paneth, Program in Epidemiology, MSU; Michaela Zint and James Dearing, Department of Communication, MSU; Robert Wyss, School of Journalism, MSU; and Sharon Dunwoody, Department of Journalism, University of Wisconsin-Madison.

A cross-section of Michigan news reporters participated on a Media Advisory Committee and in focus groups to review the handbook concept, format, and drafts. Their advice has been essential to the present content and appearance of the handbook. These reporters were: Jeff Alexander, *Muskegon Chronicle*, Steve Asplund, WLCU-TV 6, Negaunee; Karl Bates, *Ann Arbor News,* Kevin Carpenter, WJRT-TV 12, Flint; Henry Erb, WOOD-TV, Grand Rapids; Cari Draft, *Lake 'n' Trail Magazine,* Merlin Dumbrille, WTCM Radio, Traverse City; Nancy Ross-Flanigan, *Detroit Free Press;* Oscar Frenette, WJR Radio, Detroit; Sue Grulke, *Alpena News,* Jerry Hodak, WJBK-TV 2, Detroit; Lynn Jarvis, *The News Herald News*, Southgate; Eric Jhylla, WNEM-TV, Saginaw; Doug Johnson, Michigan Public Radio, MSU; Jon King, WTWR Radio, Monroe; Denis Knickerbocker, *Lansing State Journal;* Mike Magner, Newhouse Newspapers; David Maurer, WSGW-WIOG Radio, Saginaw; Roger McCoy, WILX-TV,

Lansing; Dave Paulson, Booth Newspapers; Donovan Reynolds, WKAR-TV, MSU; and Leanne Trebilcock, *Manistique Pioneer-Tribune*. Many other journalists responded to written surveys.

This handbook was made possible with funding from the Michigan Great Lakes Protection Fund, through the Office of the Great Lakes, Michigan Department of Natural Resources.

MARTHA WALTER

Editor

1 RISK ASSESSMENT BASICS

Understanding how risk assessments are done is key to understanding their results, interpreting them for your audience, and detecting bogus, overblown, minimized, or unsubstantiated claims.

Key Questions to Ask about Risk Assessments

(numbers indicate pages where more information can be found)

Risk

What is the risk and type of harm from the substance in question
to the population in question? **3, 14**

What are the upper and lower limits of the risk—the range of
feasible probabilities? **3, 10**

Why does the scientist/official/interest group choose to publicize
the single risk figure given? [*If a single figure is reported.*] **10**

Data Used

How was exposure assessed? **6, 17**

How was toxicity assessed? **7, 31**

What models and assumptions were used in the exposure and
toxicity studies? **23, 24, 40, 41**

Data Not Used

What data gaps and knowledge gaps existed? **9, 18, 21, 24, 37, 40**

What assumptions were made to cover these gaps? **22, 24, 40**

How confident is the scientist that the assumptions accurately
reflect reality?

Should some of the assumptions be verified in another study?

Did study constraints require the use of non-standard methodolo-
gies or analytical techniques?

Comparisons

How does this risk compare with the risk of a similar substance,
a substance from a similar source, or an alternative or substitute
substance? [*Don't settle for a comparison with a risk people take
voluntarily, such as skiing or sky-diving.*] **91, 92**

Risk Management/Trade-Offs

What are the benefits derived from the production or use of this
substance?

What are the economic and social costs of eliminating/regulating
this substance?

Who else can I talk to?

What is Risk Assessment?

Risk assessment is a scientific process of evaluating the adverse effects caused by a substance, activity, lifestyle, or natural phenomenon.

In this handbook, *risk assessment* refers to the process of estimating the type and magnitude of risk to human health posed by exposure to chemical substances.

Assessments of environmental human health risks combine information on the amount of a substance humans are exposed to and the *toxicity* of that substance in order to state what is likely to happen.

Risk assessment is characterized by uncertainty. Although scientists have learned much about environmental contaminants, limited data and knowledge still require researchers to make assumptions throughout the risk assessment process.

The results of a risk assessment should report what assumptions were made as well as the type of harm and its magnitude.

The uncertainty inherent in risk assessment means that risk assessors cannot precisely describe the risk. Rather, they should state the range of probabilities which they found.

Ideally, risk assessments are science-based estimates of the human health risk faced by a population exposed to a particular substance. The risk should be stated as a range of probabilities.

Example of risk stated as a range of probabilities: "Our best estimate of the risk of cancer from chemical X is one additional case in 10,000 people, but the risk could be as high as one additional case in 1,000 people, or as low as no additional cases."

The Steps in Risk Assessment

A risk assessment consists of four steps.

❑ *Problem Identification. What substances should be tested?* Every natural or manmade substance cannot be tested at once, due to limited resources. Scientists and regulatory agencies must identify for study those substances that apparently cause health problems in humans.

❑ *Exposure Assessment. How much of a substance are people actually exposed to?* Once a suspect substance is identified, scientists conduct studies to estimate the amount of the substance a particular population is exposed to.

❑ *Toxicity Assessment. How much of the substance causes what kind of harm to humans?* Scientists also study the type and degree of harm different amounts of the substance cause in humans.

❑ *Risk Characterization. What is the risk posed by this substance in its present (or predicted) use patterns?* In risk characterization, scientists combine information from exposure assessments and toxicity assessments to estimate the type and magnitude of risk faced by the exposed population. The risk characterization should also state areas of uncertainty in the exposure and toxicity assessments that may affect the outcome.

Risk assessments combine information on the level of exposure to a substance and its toxicity to characterize what is likely to happen to humans who may be exposed.

The Steps in Risk Assessment (cont.)

Problem Identification

The problem identification step evaluates whether a substance may cause harm.

Scientific or public concerns about harm from a particular substance often initiate the problem identification process.

Direct evidence of harm to humans is seldom available. Instead, evidence is gathered by:

- ❏ **animal studies.** If the substance causes health problems in animals, it is assumed that it *may* be harmful to humans. Animal studies are the most common type of problem identification study.

- ❏ ***in vitro* (test tube) studies.** Experiments on isolated cells or microorganisms are used to explore how chemicals may exert toxic effects.

- ❏ **comparison studies.** The properties of the substance in question are compared with substances known to be harmful. (In vitro and comparison studies are less conclusive than animal studies, but they can augment them.)

- ❏ **epidemiological studies.** If available, these provide the most reliable evidence. However, their relevance to the present population of concern (perhaps a particularly sensitive one such as children) must be judged.

Ideally, if a substance is found to be possibly harmful to humans, it will be further studied in exposure and toxicity assessments.

Problem identification is performed to judge whether a substance may cause harm to humans, usually by looking at the effect of the substance on animals.

The Steps in Risk Assessment (cont.)

Exposure Assessment

The *exposure assessment* step estimates how much of a substance a population inhales, ingests, or absorbs through the skin.

Long-term exposures to chemicals in the environment are usually assessed by *environmental exposure studies*. These estimate the amount of the substance in the environment; then estimate how much of it people take in.

Some of the factors an exposure assessment must consider are:

- ❑ how long people have been exposed.
- ❑ whether the exposure was continuous or intermittent.
- ❑ how they were exposed—inhalation, ingestion, or absorption through the skin.

Again, many uncertainties may enter into these measurements, given incomplete knowledge of:

- ❑ how chemicals behave in the environment.
- ❑ people's lifestyles and how these affect exposure.

An exposure assessment should describe the uncertainties present.

The Steps in Risk Assessment (cont.)

Toxicity Assessment

The *toxicity assessment* step looks at how much of a substance causes what kind of harm to humans.

Toxicity to humans is not usually measured directly by intentionally exposing people, for obvious ethical reasons. Rather it is determined indirectly, usually by *extrapolation** of animal studies to humans.

Toxicity assessments estimate how much of a substance does what kind of harm.

The extrapolation process is one of the areas in risk assessment where many assumptions must be made. These may include assumptions about:

❐ the effects of size and biological differences between animals and humans.

❐ the effects of high doses fed the test animals versus the low doses humans usually encounter in their environment.

A toxicity assessment should describe the assumptions used and indicate the uncertainties inherent in these assumptions.

In some cases, epidemiological studies may also be used for toxicity assessment (see Chapter 4).

---

* extrapolation: the process of estimating or inferring something by extending or projecting known information, often by mathematical equations.

The Steps in Risk Assessment (cont.)

Risk Characterization

The *risk characterization* step combines the information on toxicity and exposure to describe what is likely to happen to people.

Ideally, the risk assessor has access to several toxicity and exposure studies. The risk assessor analyzes the sum total of information from these studies to develop the best possible judgment of risk.

Part of the risk assessor's job is to review the assumptions and uncertainties in the different studies and how they may have affected the study findings.

In the end, the risk assessor provides an estimate of risk, along with a description of the uncertainties that cause his/her report to be a "best guess," not an irrefutable statement of fact.

The estimate of risk is usually referred to as a "risk assessment." So the term "risk assessment" refers to both the entire process of estimating risk— problem identification, exposure assessment, toxicity assessment, and risk characterization—and to the estimate itself.

Uncertainty Unavoidable

Uncertainties are involved in all steps of a risk assessment, particularly in the toxicity assessment and the exposure assessment.

❏ In the exposure assessment, uncertainties arise because it is difficult to measure the amount of a pollutant in the environment over time, and how much is taken in by individuals.

❏ In the toxicity assessment, uncertainties arise when the findings are extrapolated from animals to humans.

Combining these uncertainties in the risk characterization step leads to a statement of risk that is not necessarily a statement of fact. However, it does indicate whether a substance may be of concern. The combined evidence of several studies is required before a statement of risk can be made with reasonable reliability.

The uncertainties inherent in risk assessments imply that a statement of risk is not necessarily a statement of absolute fact.

Results of Risk Assessments

The uncertainty inherent in risk assessment means that the risk assessors cannot precisely describe the risk. But they can and should describe the limits of the risk—how low to how high it could possibly be.

Scientists, regulators, and interest groups may describe risk as a single estimate or probability (e.g., 1 case in 10,000), rather than as a range of likely probabilities.

Anyone stating a single probability may have a variety of motivations:

❏ Scientists or other experts may state the probability that appears most likely.

❏ Officials charged to protect public health may state the higher limit of risk, or give the range in a statement that emphasizes the higher limit: "The risk can be as high as [x], but may be much lower."

❏ Individuals, organizations, or others with special interests may report only the highest or only the lowest limit, depending on the point they wish to make.

Risk assessors should describe risk as a range— from how low to how high it could be.

Example of reporting risk as a range: In a report on asbestos, the National Academy of Sciences stated that the risk of lung cancer in non-smoking males from asbestos levels commonly found in air is 6 additional cases for every million men exposed. However, they also indicated that the risk could be as low as zero or as high as 22 additional cases per million men exposed.

What Risk Assessment is Not

Sometimes a study is represented as a risk assessment when it is not.

❐ A report on the incidence of cancer to rats from a certain substance is not a risk assessment. It only defines the toxicity to rats.

❐ An extrapolation of this information to the incidence of cancer in humans at postulated levels of exposure is a toxicity assessment, not a risk assessment.

❐ Risk assessment occurs only when information from toxicity assessments is combined with information from exposure assessments (how much of the substance people are actually exposed to).

Ideally, the risk assessment describes what is likely to happen to a particular population under real world conditions.

Risk assessments are based on estimates of both exposure and toxicity. Ideally, they describe what is likely to happen to a particular population under real world conditions.

Risk Assessment versus Risk Management

Risk assessment is distinct from risk management.

Risk assessment is a scientific process of investigating phenomena to estimate the level of risk.

Risk management is an effort to reduce the risk through education, regulation, and clean-up.

Risk managers use the results of risk assessments, plus economic, social, and legal considerations to make regulatory and policy decisions.

While economic, social, and legal considerations have a legitimate place in risk management, they have no place in the scientific process of risk assessment.

Risk management attempts to reduce the risk that has been discovered through risk assessment.

Example of risk management: Scientists study the effects of chemical X on rats and find that adverse effects do occur. They also find that when the rats are given up to 10 grams of the chemical, there are no adverse effects.

Risk managers then use this highest no-effect value—10 grams—to determine an acceptable level of chemical X in humans. This would likely be done by dividing one or more safety factors into 10 grams. If the safety factor were 100, this would yield 0.1 gram as the acceptable level in humans.

Risk managers then use the acceptable level value to set standards. For example, they may use the value to set the maximum amount of chemical X that will be allowed in drinking water, so that no more than 0.1 gram accumulates in human tissue. By establishing these limits, risks from chemical X in drinking water will be reduced, if not eliminated.

Important Characteristics of Risk Assessments

Although economic, social, and legal factors should not figure in risk assessment, risk assessment is not completely devoid of what might be termed policy decisions.

The choices of models, data, assumptions, and methodology may be scientifically based; yet different scientists may make different decisions.

These decisions are sometimes "logical" in that they explore assumptions, data, methodology, etc. previously unexplored.

Sometimes they are intuitive—based on the scientist's best judgment.

Sometimes they are influenced by external considerations, (e.g., the public's great fear of cancer may influence researchers to select worst-case models of how cancers are formed).

These decisions affect the outcome of the risk assessment, although they are often not described.

Reporters can get a clearer view of a risk assessment by asking about the choices the scientist made—models, data, assumptions, and methodology.

Figure 1: Basics of Environmental Risk Assessment

EXPOSURE ASSESSMENT

WHAT IT DOES:

Estimates the amount of a substance a population is exposed to.

HOW IT'S DONE:

Measures:
amount in environment.
amount in human tissue.
Employs:
models of chemical behavior.
models of human behavior.

THE RESULTS ARE:

Amount of the substance ingested, inhaled, or absorbed per unit of time by the exposed population.
Example: "An average person in community X is exposed to 50-150 mg/day of substance Y through eating, drinking, and breathing."

TOXICITY ASSESSMENT

WHAT IT DOES:

Estimates the toxicity of a substance to humans.

HOW IT'S DONE:

non-carcinogenic toxicity. Uses animal studies.
carcinogenic toxicity. Uses epidemiology and animal studies called carcinogenesis bioassays.

THE RESULTS ARE:

non-carcinogenic toxicity: The maximum safe dose. *Example: "The maximum safe level of substance Y is 1 mg/kg/day."*
carcinogenic toxicity: The likelihood of disease per dose. *Example: "There will be an estimated 3 cancers per 100 people exposed to 1 mg/kg/day of substance Y for a lifetime."*

RISK ASSESSMENT

WHAT IT DOES:

Combines the results of exposure assessments and toxicity assessments to yield the risk posed to a particular population by the amount of substance that population is exposed to.

THE RESULTS ARE:

non-carcinogenic risk: Compares the exposure to the safe level.
Example: "The amount of substance Y in the community's drinking water is 4 ppm, one-half the regulatory safe level of 8 ppm."

carcinogenic risk: Gives the estimated increase in cancer rates in the exposed population. *Example: "The estimated cancer risk to population X is one additional case per 10,000 people."*

2 EXPOSURE ASSESSMENT BASICS

Before there can be a risk assessment, there must be exposure assessment. Assessing how much of a substance people are exposed to is often difficult and based partially on assumptions. The reporter who knows what assumptions have been made can ascertain how much confidence to place in an exposure estimate.

Key Questions to Ask about Exposure Assessments

(numbers indicate pages where more information can be found)

General

How much of the substance are/were people exposed to? **25**

How did the scientist measure the exposure? **19**

Personal Exposure Studies

How was the analysis done? [e.g., analysis of urine, blood, or tissue] **20**

Could any of the substance have left the body by the time measurements were made? **20**

In what other bodily fluids or tissue might this substance accumulate that were not measured? **20**

Environmental Exposure Studies

How did the scientist measure the amount of the substance in the environment? [from what sources, over what period of time, in what environmental medium—air, water, soil, or food] **22**

What assumptions did the scientist make in arriving at this figure? [e.g., number and distance of sources, behavior of substance, length of time before substance breaks down] **23**

In what ways might this substance get into the environment that the scientist didn't measure? [e.g., local or distant air emissions, intentional or accidental discharges into streams, leaking landfills, etc.] **22**

How did the scientist estimate people's exposure? [e.g., route of intake, amount taken in, length of time exposed, how an exposure measured for a studied population was extrapolated to a larger or different group] **24**

Did the scientist take into account people whose lifestyles may give them greater exposure? [e.g., factory workers, groups who live closer to the source, ethnic or income groups with different diets, etc.] **24**

Exposure Assessment Overview

Exposure assessment is a major component of risk assessment.*

An exposure assessment evaluates how much of a substance an individual or population ingests, inhales, or contacts through the skin over a period of time.

Exposure may be long-term or short-term and occupational or environmental. Exposure is most frequently assessed by *environmental exposure studies*. These studies:

❏ estimate how much of a substance is/was present in the environment and how much of it people actually come/came into contact with.

❏ are usually conducted to assess long-term exposures.†

Exposure can also be assessed by *personal exposure studies*. These studies analyze bodily fluids or tissues to calculate how much of a substance people are exposed to.

An exposure assessment evaluates how much of a substance people come into contact with, how often, and for how long a period.

---

* Other components are toxicity assessment (Chapter 3) and problem identification and risk characterization (Chapter 1).

† Ideally, scientists would like to know the amount of chemical that gets to the site in the body where toxicity occurs. Since this is not possible in most cases, the amount that the individual is in contact with is used as the measure of exposure. Exposure can lead to either local effects (burns, rashes, etc.) as a result of direct contact, or to systemic (whole body) effects when it is absorbed into the bloodstream.

Exposure Classifications

Exposures are usually classified as either long-term or short-term and as either occupational or environmental.

- **Occupational exposures** are generally easier to measure, because they occur in a confined space during known lengths of time.

- **Environmental exposures** involve greater uncertainty. The individual may be exposed to a chemical in a variety of locations—home, traffic, shopping—and for varying amounts of time. The great mobility of people in modern society adds to the complexity of this determination.

Exposures are classified as long-term or short-term and as occupational or environmental.

Examples of exposures:

- **Long-term, occupational exposure:** A factory worker inhales a chemical eight hours a day, five days a week, over several years.

- **Short-term, occupational exposure:** A plant explosion creates fumes that workers inhale for a few minutes.

- **Long-term, environmental exposure:** People in a community drink water from wells contaminated by seepage from an industrial disposal site.

- **Short-term environmental exposure:**
  - A child eats 10 aspirin in 5 minutes.
  - People in several city blocks breathe fumes for a few hours after a train tank car spills a hazardous substance.

Measuring Exposure

Exposure can be estimated in two ways.

- *Personal exposure studies* measure the amounts of a substance in the body.

  This method is usually appropriate after a short-term exposure, when the full amount of the substance taken in may still be in the body.

- *Environmental exposure studies* measure amounts of a substance in the environment, determine the route of exposure (inhalation, ingestion, or skin contact), and estimate how much is in contact with the population.

  This method is usually appropriate for measuring long-term exposures to substances that the human body breaks down and excretes. However, variability over time in the concentration of the substance in the environment may lead to uncertainty in this type of study.

Exposures are estimated in two ways—directly by measuring body fluids or tissues or indirectly by analyzing environmental levels of contaminants.

Examples of exposure studies:

- **Personal exposure study:** If someone is suffering from the symptoms associated with lead poisoning, the blood can be tested to determine if lead is present and at what level.

- **Environmental exposure study:** If an incinerator emits a chemical of concern, calculations can be performed to estimate the amount inhaled by an individual at a particular distance and direction from the incinerator.

*Personal exposures
are usually measured
by analyzing bodily
fluids or tissues.*

Measuring Exposure (cont.)

Personal Exposure Studies

Personal exposure is usually measured by analyzing bodily tissues or fluids. Such measures may detect:

- **Presence** of a substance.
  - Recent exposure may be detected through blood or urine tests.
  - Past exposure may be detected through analysis of tissues such as fat and bone. For example, some *organic chemicals,* which are stored in fat, can be detected this way.
- **Bodily changes** that indicate a substance is or was present.
  - Some chemicals leave the body quickly, but cause physiological changes. For example, certain pesticides change the level of an enzyme in the blood. By measuring the magnitude of change, scientists can estimate how much pesticide the person was exposed to.

Measuring Exposure (cont.)

Environmental Exposure Studies

When conducting environmental exposure studies, scientists:

- ❒ measure or estimate the amount of the substance present in the environment—air, soil, water, food;

- ❒ then estimate how much of the substance people are exposed to—ingested, inhaled, or in skin contact with—using available data, models, and assumptions.

Both of the above steps include uncertainties because of incomplete knowledge about the properties of chemical substances, their behavior in the environment, how these substances and humans interact, and the variability in personal lifestyles.

In environmental exposure studies, scientists measure the amount of substance present, then estimate how much of it people are in contact with.

It is most difficult to assess exposures from environmental contaminants when they are from distant or multiple sources or are present over a long time.

Measuring Exposure (cont.)

Environmental Exposure Studies (cont.)

AMOUNT OF SUBSTANCE IN ENVIRONMENT

Measuring the amount of a substance in the environment is usually straightforward for short-term exposures. Estimating long-term past exposures is usually more complex.

Long-term estimates are difficult when:

- all the sources are hard to identify.
- the exact emissions of all sources over time may not be known.
- movement of the substance is difficult to assess. For example, wind direction, rainfall, or groundwater seepage may be difficult to measure over time.
- the sources vary over time. For example, if the substance is in a food item, the amount may vary according to maturity, season, or other factors.

Examples of measuring long-term exposures:

- Substances in drinking water can be measured, and if past measurements are available, scientists will know the amount present over time.
- If measurements were not made previously, scientists must estimate the amount that was present. Commonly they determine the source of the substance, and estimate how much was emitted and for how long. Then they use mathematical models to calculate how much entered the medium (drinking water, air, soil, food) that people were exposed to.
- There may be many sources. For mercury in fish, there may be both local and distant sources, such as different industries. Scientists identify the sources and use mathematical models to calculate transport and estimate the amount present in fish over time.

Measuring Exposure (cont.)

Environmental Exposure Studies *(cont.)*

MODELS

The *mathematical models* used to calculate the movement of chemicals are based on the properties of the chemical in question. These properties include:

❏ vapor pressure—how easily it evaporates.

❏ solubility—how easily it dissolves in different mediums, such as water or animal fat.

❏ adsorption—how strongly it attaches to soil.

❏ persistence—how rapidly it is broken down in the environment.

Exposure models are based on chemical properties.

Examples of chemical properties:

❏ Benzene evaporates readily and breaks down quickly in the air. However, it is soluble in water and does not adsorb to soil readily. Thus, if it leaks or is poured onto the ground, it is likely to be found in groundwater, where it may reach humans through the water supply.

❏ Toxaphene evaporates slowly, but once in the air it is very persistent and is also persistent in animals. Thus, it can be deposited in distant lakes and bioaccumulated through the aquatic food chain, reaching people through the fish.

❏ PCBs dissolve only slightly in water, but a much larger amount will dissolve in the fat of living things. Thus, eating fish containing PCBs would expose someone to more PCBs than drinking the water the fish came from.

AMOUNT OF EXPOSURE

After the amount of the substance in the environment is assessed, the route of exposure must be determined—inhalation, ingestion, or skin contact—and the amount that people take in is then estimated.

Incomplete knowledge of human behavior requires that assumptions must be made to estimate how much of the chemical is taken in. Scientists must make assumptions about such things as:

- how much water or a specific food do people drink or eat each day.
- whether people filter their water/how they prepare their food.
- how much time people spend indoors/outdoors.
- whether behaviors vary with age, socio-economic class, or ethnic group.

Scientists have to characterize people's behavior to estimate exposure.

Example of the effect of different behaviors: Subsistence fishers, such as Native Americans of the Great Lakes region and some urban poor, have a higher proportion of fish in their diet than sport fishers or restaurant and fish market customers. As the decline of contaminants in fish continues, the level of safety for subsistence fishers may be achieved later than for other fish consumers.

Statements of Exposure

An exposure assessment is stated in terms of the likelihood that people are exposed to a given level of a substance over a specified period of time.

Uncertainty will be intrinsic in the assessment because of the assumptions that were made. Thus the exposure assessment should be reported as a range of exposures.

In order to protect especially sensitive groups, those responsible for protecting health may base their decisions and statements on the highest feasible exposure in the range.

This highest exposure value may be quite different from the value that scientists believe to be the best estimate of exposure to the hypothetical "average" person.

The exposure should be stated as a range of possible exposures.

Example of an exposure assessment: Groundwater that is used for drinking water is found to have nitrate at 10 ppm (10 mg/liter). A person drinking 2 liters of the water each day will have an exposure of 20 mg/day from this source. Nitrates are also found in food, and the average person consumes about 75 mg of nitrate each day from this source. Thus, if drinking water and food are the only sources of nitrate, the total exposure for this individual would be 95 mg/day. However, daily water consumption varies and the water may come from a variety of sources. In addition, an individual may eat foods that are higher or lower in nitrate than the average. Thus, the total exposure is better described as a range from 50 mg/day to 250 mg/day.

Once an exposure assessment estimates the level of exposure, scientists can apply the results of toxicity assessments to estimate the degree of harm to the exposed population.

Role of Exposure Assessment in Risk Assessment

In the end, an exposure assessment provides information on how much of a substance a population has been or will be exposed to.

An exposure assessment enables the results of toxicity assessments to be applied to the real world. That is, once the exposure assessment has estimated the amount of a substance the population of interest has actually been exposed to, then the results of the toxicity assessments can be used to estimate the degree of harm to that population.

This task is conducted by the risk assessor. The risk assessor is most often an individual trained in toxicology, the study of toxic substances. However, risk assessments may be done by scientists with other skills or by teams of scientists—some expert in environmental distribution and fate and others in toxicology.

3 TOXICITY ASSESSMENT BASICS

Before there can be a risk assessment, there must be toxicity assessments. Scientists use different procedures to assess toxicity, depending on whether they are looking for carcinogenic or non-carcinogenic effects. Awareness of these procedures will help reporters ask questions to clarify the significance and relevance of a toxicity assessment.

Key Questions to Ask About Toxicity Assessments

(numbers indicate pages where more information can be found)

Toxicity

How toxic is the substance to humans? **29**

What are the effects, precisely? **29, 30**

What type of studies were conducted to reach these conclusions? **31**

Have there been other toxicity assessments of this substance? If so, did they use different animals, methods, or models? What did they find?

Route of Exposure

Were the test animals exposed to the substance by the same route by which people are exposed? [ingesting, inhaling, absorbing through skin]

If not, has this difference been accounted for?

Models/Safety Factors

What model or safety factor was used to extrapolate the experimental results to humans? **36, 40**

Why was this model or safety factor chosen? **37, 41**

Are other models or safety factors viewed as valid by some scientists or officials?

Other Effects

Is the toxicity of this substance altered by other substances people are exposed to?

Is the substance harmful to animals, fish, or birds in the environment?

Does this substance have other harmful effects? Does it have beneficial effects? What are these effects?

Toxicity Assessment Overview

Toxicity assessment is a major component of risk assessment.*

A toxicity assessment is a tool to investigate the potential for a substance to cause harm—and how much causes what kind of harm.

All substances are toxic in quantity. Many therapeutic medications are acutely toxic, but beneficial when used at the appropriate level. Vitamin D, table salt, oxygen, and water are toxic in quantity. Thus, the mere presence of a substance does not automatically imply harm. This is why toxicity assessment is concerned with the type and degree of harm caused by differing amounts of a substance.

There is no one measure of toxicity. Effects may occur in the short term (acute effects) or after repeated exposures over a long time (chronic effects). They may affect only one part of the body or many, and they may vary greatly in severity.†

A toxicity assessment provides an estimate of how much of a substance causes what kind of harm.

---

* Other components are exposure assessment (Chapter 2) and hazard identification and risk characterization (Chapter 1).

† The term *toxicity* refers to the inherent potential of a substance to cause systemic damage to living organisms. The term *hazardous* is very different. It refers to the potential of a substance to (1) cause any of several kinds of harm, through toxicity, flammability, explosiveness, corrosiveness etc., and (2) the ease with which people can come in contact with it. Hazardous is not a synonym for toxic.

Toxic Effects

Toxic effects are classified as either acute or chronic.

- ❑ **Acute effects** happen very rapidly after a single exposure has occurred (food poisoning, breathing fumes from a chlorine spill). Sweating, nausea, paralysis, and death are examples of acute effects.

- ❑ **Chronic effects** happen only after repeated long-term exposure (cigarette smoking, eating foods with low levels of contaminants, breathing polluted air). Cancer, organ damage, reproductive difficulties, and nervous system impairment are examples of chronic effects.

These chronic effects fall into two categories: carcinogenic effects and non-carcinogenic effects.

There are two types of toxic effects— acute and chronic.

Examples of non-carcinogenic chronic effects:

- ❑ **Organ damage:** cirrhosis of the liver from long-term alcohol consumption; emphysema from long-term tobacco smoking.

- ❑ **Reproductive difficulty:** decreased fertility from the pesticide DBCP (dibromochloropropane).

- ❑ **Nervous system impairment:** mental retardation in people exposed to high levels of lead during early childhood.

Assessing Toxicity

All quantitative toxicity assessments are based on the *dose-response* concept: as you increase the dose (exposure), the response (toxicity) also increases.

Scientists perform studies to determine exactly how high a dose causes what kind of a response, or effect. The smaller the dose needed to cause an effect, the more potent (toxic) the substance is.

For all compounds other than cancer-causing agents (carcinogens), it is assumed that there is a dose below which no effect occurs (a *threshold*). This is similar to a drug where too small of a dose has no beneficial effect.

For carcinogens, it is often assumed that even the smallest dose can cause an effect (no threshold) (see page 41).

Although the dose-response concept is used in all types of toxicity assessments, it is used somewhat differently for each of them.

Acute toxic effects are estimated by LD_{50} studies or observation of accidental exposures (see pages 32-33).

Chronic toxic effects are estimated by dose-response studies on animals (pages 35-37). **Carcinogenic effects** are estimated by a type of dose-response study called a *carcinogenesis bioassay* (pages 38-41).

The dose-response concept is the basis for all toxicity assessments. It is used differently to evaluate acute effects and chronic effects.

Assessing Acute Toxicity

Acute toxicity is assessed using observations of accidental human exposures or by conducting LD_{50} tests on experimental animals, usually rodents.

Most information about *acute toxicity* of chemicals to humans comes from accidental poisonings or exposures, such as drug overdoses or chemical spills. Physicians/researchers know or estimate the level of exposure and observe and document the effects.

Scientists also use animal tests called LD_{50} (L-D-fifty) studies to assess acute toxicity. These studies determine the amount of a substance that will kill half the test animals in 14 days. This amount is called the LD_{50}—Lethal Dose for 50% of the animals.

LD_{50} is stated in milligrams per kilogram (mg/kg): milligram of chemical per kilogram of body weight.

The lower the LD_{50}—the lower the lethal dose—the more toxic the substance.

Example: A reported "rat oral LD_{50} of 50 mg/kg" means that half of the rats that ingested a dose of 50 milligrams of the substance per kilogram of body weight died within 14 days.

* The term LC_{50}—Lethal Concentration—is used to measure the toxicity of gases. The LC_{50} is stated in milligram of chemical per liter (or cubic meter) of air.

Assessing Acute Toxicity (cont.)

LD_{50} values are unknown for humans, since LD_{50} experiments are not conducted on humans. If a LD_{50} statement is applied to humans, it must in actuality be either:

❑ an animal LD_{50}.

❑ the "average lethal dose" (ALD), calculated from the effects of accidental poisonings and exposures. Also called mean lethal dose (MLD).

❑ the "lethal amount" calculated from an animal LD_{50}. This calculation is done by multiplying the LD_{50} by a number representing average human weight.

LD_{50} values are unknown for humans, but animal LD_{50} values can be used to estimate lethal amounts for humans.

Example of lethal amount: If the LD_{50} is 50 mg/kg:

The lethal amount for a child would be 50 mg/kg times 10 kg, which equals 500 mg (about 1/8 tsp.)

The lethal amount for an adult would be 50 mg/kg times 70 kg, which is 3,500 mg (about 3/4 tsp.)*

---

*The 10 kg and 70 kg in the example above come from the weight of the "average" person—10 kg (22 lbs) for a child; 70 kg (154 lbs) for an adult.

Assessing Chronic Toxicity

Chronic toxicity can be divided into two categories:

- ❏ cancer (carcinogenic toxicity).
- ❏ all other effects (non-carcinogenic toxicity).

Cancer is in a separate category because public concern about it is so great. People want to know if even one person in a million persons who are exposed to a substance will get cancer. To discover this, researchers conduct a specific type of dose-response study—a *carcinogenesis bioassay* (see pages 38-41).

Non-carcinogenic effects are usually assessed with a different type of dose-response study (see following pages).

Non-Carcinogenic Assessment

Introduction

Scientists assess non-carcinogenic chronic toxicity by administering varying amounts of a substance (dose) to laboratory animals and noting the effects (responses), if any, at each dose.

Essentially, the scientists look for the smallest dose that causes any detectable effect. This smallest dose is called the *Lowest Observable Effect Level (LOEL).* *

To conduct these dose-response studies, scientists:

- ❏ Administer different small doses of a substance to several groups of test animals every day over a lifetime.

- ❏ Periodically examine and finally autopsy the animals to determine if any effects have occurred. The effects may be:

  - ❏ damage to an organ,

  - ❏ behavioral modifications,

  - ❏ change in the level of an essential body chemical.

- ❏ Determine the smallest dose at which an effect occurs—the Lowest Observable Effect Level (LOEL).†

- ❏ LOEL is measured in milligrams (mg) of substance per kilogram (kg) of body weight, or in parts per million (ppm) of substance in food.

Non-carcinogenic chronic toxicity is assessed by studies to determine the smallest dose that causes any detectable effect.

3

---

* In addition to LOEL, the term LOAEL (Lowest Observable Adverse Effect Level) is sometimes used. The term LOAEL implies a judgment that the effect is adverse. A LOEL refers to any effect and may or may not be judged to be adverse.

† This dose may still be a high dose compared to environmental exposures.

Determining Safe Levels

When performing the experiments just described, scientists also determine the highest dose at which no effects occur—the *No Observable Effect Level (NOEL).**

The NOEL is considered the "safe level" for that chemical in the species studied.

The NOEL is not necessarily the "safe level" for humans, because:

❑ humans may be more/less sensitive to the substance than the animals studied.

❑ humans have more genetic, health, age, and other variabilities, which may affect individual human reactions.†

To account for these differences, public health officials divide the NOEL by a safety factor, usually 100, to arrive at a presumed "safe level" for humans. If the NOEL for a substance were 100 mg/kg, the "safe level" for humans would be considered 1 mg/kg.

This "safe level" is most likely lower than scientists' best estimate of the NOEL in humans. However, it is the number risk managers use to establish regulations, such as the maximum amount of a chemical allowed in drinking water, and to create guidelines such as fish consumption advisories.

> *To protect the public, scientists also determine the highest dose at which no effects occur.*

---

* The term No Observable Adverse Effect Level (NOAEL) is sometimes used. The term NOAEL implies a judgment that the effect is adverse. A NOEL refers to any effect and may or may not be judged to be adverse.

† Lab animals are bred to be similar to one another, and an experiment will be conducted on animals of the same age and health.

Non-Carcinogenic Assessment (cont.)

Human Sensitivity and Variability

Dividing the NOEL by a safety factor assumes that humans are more sensitive than animals. But humans are not always more sensitive. For some substances, they may be less sensitive, or less sensitive than some species.

This variation is usually due to the different degrees and rates of absorption, metabolism, and/or excretion of the substance by the different species.

Although it might be reasoned that the most humanlike animals—monkeys—would be the best test animals, they react to some substances more differently from humans than other animals. For example, dogs react to nitrobenzene similarly to humans, while monkeys do not.

Knowledge is still incomplete regarding the best test animals for different types of substances and whether humans can be expected to be more or less sensitive to any particular compound.

The "safe level" calculation for humans assumes that humans are more sensitive than animals, but humans are not more sensitive in all cases.

Examples of human sensitivity:

- ❑ **More sensitivity:** The drug Thalidomide caused no adverse effects in the animals studied, but caused severe birth defects in humans.

- ❑ **Less sensitivity:** Insecticides are often developed to be more toxic to insects than to humans. Since people are less sensitive to these chemicals, they can use them without injuring themselves.

- ❑ **Genetic variability:** People vary widely in their reactions to bee venom. Some show almost no reaction to a bee sting; others may die without immediate medical treatment.

Carcinogenesis Bioassay

Introduction

Scientists assess carcinogenic toxicity very differently than they assess non-carcinogenic toxicity. This is in response to public fear about cancer.

People want to know if even one in a million individuals will get cancer from exposure to a suspected carcinogen. To find this out with any degree of confidence by traditional dose-response studies, scientists would have to use several million test animals. The impracticality of such experiments has led to the development of the *carcinogenesis bioassay.**

With a carcinogenesis bioassay, scientists are not looking for the safe level of exposure (NOEL). Rather, harm is assumed, and they are looking for the incidence, or risk, of harm.

---

* The carcinogesis bioassay is a method of testing substances for carcinogenic effects that utilizes high-dose studies on laboratory animals to look for even the rare case of cancer. It is not necessarily the best scientific approach to assess the carcinogenic effects of chemicals. Instead it is a way to respond to public concerns by generating carcinogenic risk values with large margins of safety.

Carcinogenesis Bioassay (cont.)

Methodology

Scientists assess carcinogenic toxicity by feeding large doses of the substance in question to animals in an effort to find even the rare case of cancer resulting from exposure to it.

❑ Test animals are administered different large doses of a substance daily over a lifetime (24-30 months in rats).

❑ At the end of the study, the animals are examined to see if cancer can be found.

❑ If cancer is found, scientists use available data and *mathematical models* to:

   ❑ estimate the cancer incidence at the lower doses more likely to occur in the environment.

   ❑ estimate the effect of the size and sensitivity differences between the test animals and human beings.

To measure carcinogenic toxicity, scientists try to find even the rare case of cancer.

Example of a carcinogenesis bioassay: A carcinogenesis bioassay was performed for benzene on both rats and mice. Both sexes of each species got leukemia at the high doses administered. Extrapolating the cancer incidence at high dose to low dose and from rodents to humans resulted in the risk estimate that a benzene dose of 1 mg/kg/day will result in 3 cancers per 100 people exposed daily for a lifetime to that dose. This dose is much higher than anyone would be exposed to in the environment under normal conditions.

The choice of model has a strong influence on the outcome of the study.

Carcinogenesis Bioassay (cont.)

Mathematical Models Vary

A *mathematical model* is a set of equations that mimic a real situation and predict what will happen under different circumstances.

In toxicity assessments, scientists do not know what will happen to humans exposed to the low doses found in the environment. So models are developed to apply information gained in animal studies to the human condition. Many educated assumptions must be made in developing these models.*

The choice of model will have a strong influence on the outcome of the toxicity assessment, because when scientists apply different models to identical data, they will get different results.

---

* These assumptions regard: similarities and differences between animal and human reactions; the effects of genetic, age, health, and other variations in humans; and whether only one molecule or many molecules of a carcinogen are sufficient to start a cancer process under appropriate conditions (see next page). Since not all carcinogens work the same way, a particular type of model may give a fairly realistic risk value for some, but a very unrealistic risk value for others.

Carcinogenesis Bioassay (cont.)

Non-Threshold vs. Threshold Models

Two fundamentally different types of mathematical models are applied to carcinogenic risk assessment. One is called a *non-threshold model* and is based on the assumption that even one molecule of a cancer-causing agent can lead to the disease. This type of model is also referred to as a "one-hit" model.

The second type of mathematical model is called a *threshold model* and is based on the premise that repeated exposures to a chemical are needed before a threshold of exposure is reached and cancer follows.

Scientists in regulatory agencies generally use non-threshold models for carcinogenesis bioassays. These assign to a substance a higher estimate of cancer potency than would threshold models. (However, the threshold model is currently used to assess risk of all non-carcinogenic chemicals.)

Public health officials generally rely on non-threshold models—models that make worst-case assumptions.

Examples:

Non-Threshold (linear) Dose-Response Model

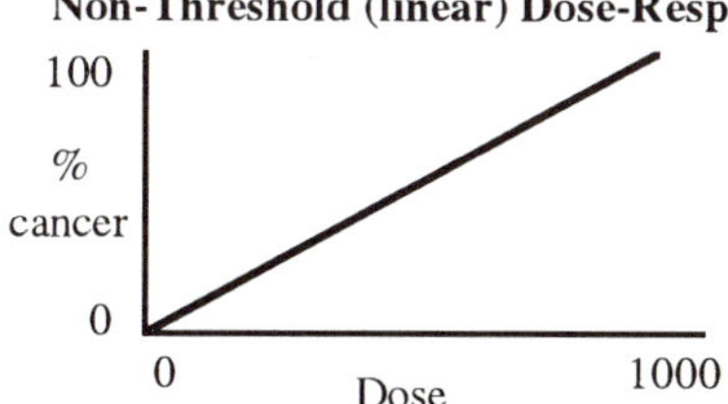

Threshhold Dose-Response Model

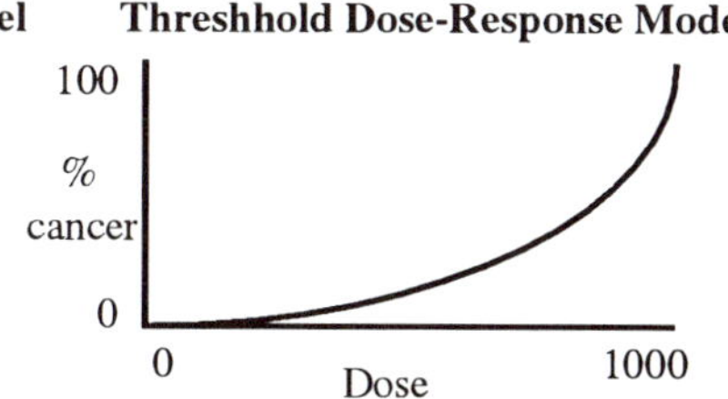

Role of Toxicity Assessment in Risk Assessment

In the end, a toxicity assessment provides information on how much of a chemical causes what kind of harm.

If the toxicity assessment is based on an animal study, the degree of harm to humans must be extrapolated using mathematical models based on a variety of assumptions. Thus the toxicity assessment provides only an estimate of the harm to humans.

As more toxicity studies on a particular chemical are conducted—dose-response studies on different species of animals for example, or epidemiological and *in vitro* (test tube) studies—scientists become more confident in their characterization of the toxicity of the substance.

The risk assessor's job is to determine the real world risk to humans of a substance by combining information on toxicity and exposure. This job is made more complicated if data are collected from many different studies, but the results will be more likely to reflect the best estimates scientists can make.

4 EPIDEMIOLOGY: THE SCIENCE OF PEOPLE

Epidemiology is the most direct method of assessing risk to humans, but like any scientific method, it has its own limitations and problems of interpretation. Knowing the principles and pitfalls of epidemiology will help you interpret epidemiological studies.

Key Questions to Ask about Epidemiological Studies

(numbers indicate pages where more information can be found)

What kind of study was conducted? [*case-control, cohort, cross-sectional, or clinical trial*] **48-52**

If a cross-sectional study, do the results indicate a possible problem requiring further study? [*Cross-sectional studies do not establish cause and effect.*] **51**

If a case-control or cohort study, what were the characteristics of the two groups being compared? **48, 49**

What characteristic(s) did the investigators identify as being associated with the disease?

Does the association between the characteristic and the disease reflect an actual cause-effect relationship? **54**

If so, on what does the investigator base that conclusion? [*e.g., strength of association, dose-response relationship, consistency, specificity, etc.*] **54**

What is the relative risk of the disease from the characteristic? **53**

What have other investigators found? **57**

What is Epidemiology?

Epidemiology is the study of patterns of disease in human *populations**. Because epidemiological studies look directly at humans rather than extrapolate from animals, they provide the most compelling evidence for measuring environmental risks to humans.

Most studies in recent decades that have linked environmental factors to human diseases were designed using principles of epidemiology.

Epidemiological studies have provided the critical evidence to link:

❏ toxic shock syndrome to tampon use.

❏ leukemia to on-the-job exposures to benzene.

❏ heart attacks to cholesterol.

❏ lung cancer, heart attacks, and low birth weight to cigarette smoking.

❏ Legionnaires' disease to contaminated cooling units.

Epidemiological studies provide evidence, not proof. Uncertainty is inherent in the tools that epidemiologists use. While the uncertainty can be very small, it can never be zero, because epidemiologists cannot be absolutely sure that the effect they see corresponds to the suspected cause.

Most recent studies that have convincingly linked environmental factors to human diseases were epidemiological studies.

---

* A population is a group about which a researcher wants to draw conclusions based on a sample.

Epidemiological Research

Epidemiologists compare two or more groups of people to determine what characteristics distinguish groups who get disease from groups who do not.

These distinguishing characteristics are then examined to determine how and why they are associated with disease.

Some of the characteristics epidemiologists look at are:

- consumption of certain foods.
- contact with bacteria, chemicals, or viruses.
- gender, race, or socioeconomic status.
- daily activities and behaviors.
- genetic background.
- metabolic characteristics, such as cholesterol level and blood pressure.

Epidemiological Research (cont.)

Risk Factors and Exposures

Epidemiologists prefer not to use the word "cause" when looking for clues to disease, because many characteristics associated with disease are not true causes.

For example, cigarette smoking is associated with heart attacks because chemicals in the smoke trigger the attacks. Race, gender, and socio-economic status also are strongly associated with heart attacks, not because they directly cause the attacks, but because they are proxies for many hard-to-define behaviors, environmental factors, and genetic factors that increase the risk of heart disease.

So epidemiologists use the term *"risk factor"* to describe anything that increases the risk of disease. Cigarettes, race, and socio-economic status all are risk factors for heart disease.

Risk factors also are called *exposures*. A person with a risk factor is said to be exposed; a person without that particular risk factor is unexposed.

(However, it is not usual to describe risk factors that are inherent characteristics of an individual, such as sex and race, as exposures.)

Epidemiologists prefer the term "risk factor" rather than "cause" to describe anything that increases the risk of disease.

4

Types of Epidemiological Studies

Epidemiologists favor two types of studies for searching out risk factors for disease, *case-control studies* and *cohort studies.*

Case-Control Studies

Epidemiologists survey a group of people with disease (cases) and a group without disease (controls) about their histories. The survey may involve direct questioning or examination of medical or other records.

The basic question: *What differs in the histories of these two groups that could explain why one is diseased and the other is not?*

Case-control studies look at the histories of cases and controls for clues to what causes disease in the cases.

Example of a case-control study: In the spring of 1980, U.S. doctors diagnosed hundreds of cases of toxic shock syndrome (TSS), a potentially fatal, previously rare disease. Most cases occurred in young women during their menstrual periods. Investigators at the Centers for Disease Control questioned 50 women with toxic shock syndrome (cases) about their use of sanitary products in the month before they got sick. Then they asked each woman for the names of three friends who did not have TSS (controls), and asked them the same questions. Women with TSS were more likely than their friends to have used tampons; in particular they were almost 8 times as likely to have used one brand: Rely. This brand was withdrawn from the market in September 1980, and the incidence of TSS decreased dramatically.

Types of Epidemiological Studies (cont.)

Cohort Studies (Follow-up Studies)

A cohort study begins with a group of people who do not have the disease being studied. Group members differ on one or more characteristics suspected of causing the disease (for example, some may smoke while others do not). The group is followed over time to see if members with the suspect characteristic are more likely to develop the disease.

The basic question: *Are the people with the suspect characteristic at greater risk of getting disease?*

Cohort studies follow groups through time to determine whether group members with a suspected risk factor are more likely to get disease.

4

Example of a cohort study: To evaluate the effect of environmental lead exposure on children's IQs, researchers followed 516 children in the lead-smelting town of Port Pirie, Australia, from birth to age seven, periodically taking blood samples to measure lead levels. At age seven, children with highest blood lead levels over the years had the lowest IQs.

*Case-control studies
are more common,
but cohort studies
are generally
more convincing.*

Types of Epidemiological Studies (cont.)

Which Kind of Study is Better?

Case-control studies are more common than cohort studies because they are faster and cheaper. Also, for relatively uncommon diseases like childhood leukemia, they often are the only practical way to look for causes of disease.

Cohort studies are more convincing for two reasons:

- they provide a much better opportunity to establish a cause-effect relationship because they begin with the exposure (cause) and move forward in time to the disease (effect). In contrast, case-control studies begin with the disease (effect) and look back to the exposure (cause). It is not always clear that the identified cause actually did come first.

- case-control studies are more prone to certain study design problems, such as bias or chance (see Chapter 5).

But cohort studies have their own drawbacks:

- they are very expensive.

- they take a long time (because they start with well people and wait for them to get sick).

- they are difficult to conduct properly because study subjects tend to drop out of the study over time.

Types of Epidemiological Studies (cont.)

Two other types of epidemiological studies—*cross-sectional studies* and *clinical trials*—are often in the news. While these studies serve valuable purposes, epidemiologists generally do not use them to investigate risk factors for disease.

Cross-Sectional Studies

The cross-sectional study identifies a population of interest (people in a particular neighborhood, people coming to a clinic) and asks its members about current diseases and current exposures.

Cross-sectional studies offer epidemiologists a quick way to determine whether a problem exists that warrants further study—whether, for example, workers in a particular industry have an unusually high rate of disease.

But this kind of study is not useful for establishing cause and effect because it is difficult to determine whether the exposures actually caused the disease.

Cross-sectional studies help identify whether a problem exists that warrants further study. They are not useful for determining cause and effect.

Example of misinterpretation from a cross-sectional study: It is well known that cigarette smoking increases the risk of a heart attack. But if researchers did not know this and surveyed a city's residents to determine who had heart disease and who smoked, they might find that healthy people smoke more than people with heart disease. The real reason for this result is that people tend to quit smoking after they are diagnosed with heart disease. (In effect, the outcome is influencing the cause.) However, to the researchers it might appear that cigarette smoking protects against heart disease. Many cross-sectional studies suffer from this chicken–egg problem.

Clinical Trials

A *clinical trial* is a study done to test the effectiveness of a drug or other treatment.

Clinical trials test the effectiveness of a drug or treatment.

Patients with a particular disease are randomly assigned to receive either the treatment under study or an inactive placebo (or the standard treatment, if one exists). Patients are then followed for a specified period to determine whether patients receiving the new treatment do better than those getting the standard treatment or the placebo.

Clinical trials are the best of epidemiological studies in terms of the quality of the information they provide. However, as a rule, they can't be used to explore causes of disease because it is unethical to assign people to be exposed to suspected toxins. However, such trials may be very useful for studying preventive measures, such as vaccines.

Example of a clinical trial: (See example on page 64.)

Estimating Risk

At the end of a study, researchers calculate the *risk ratio* or *relative risk,* by comparing the occurrence of disease in two groups—one group with a suspect characteristic, and one group without. This is the source of statements like "people who smoke are 10 times as likely to get lung cancer as people who do not."

Risk ratio close to 1 suggests the characteristic has no effect on disease.

Risk ratio greater than 1 suggests the characteristic increases risk of disease.

Risk ratio less than 1 suggests the characteristic protects against disease.

Epidemiologists use risk ratios to describe the effect a characteristic has on disease.

4

Example of risk ratios: In a landmark study, scientists followed 34,445 British male physicians from 1951 to 1961 to see if those who smoked had a higher rate of lung cancer. At the end of 10 years, the statistics looked like this:

Lung cancer death rate:

among nonsmokers:	7 per 100,000
among those smoking up to a half pack daily:	54 per 100,000
among those smoking up to a pack daily:	139 per 100,000
among those smoking more than a pack daily:	227 per 100,000

Dividing rates among smokers by the rate among nonsmokers yields ratios which show that, compared to nonsmokers:

Smokers of up to a half pack daily were almost **8 times** as likely to die of lung cancer—(54/7=7.7; the **risk ratio** was 7.7).

Smokers of up to a pack a day were almost **20 times** as likely to die of lung cancer—(139/7=19.9; the **risk ratio** was 19.9).

Smokers of more than a pack a day were more than **32 times** as likely to die of lung cancer—(227/7=32.4; the **risk ratio** was 32.4).

If the data indicate an association, the researcher must explore whether a cause-effect relation-ship truly exists.

Causation Criteria

If an *association* has been observed between an exposure and a disease, and *bias*, *confounders*, and other possible errors have been reasonably accounted for (see Chapter 5), then researchers can address the question of whether the association is likely to reflect a true cause-effect relationship. Some commonly used criteria are:

Strength of association. The exposure is associated with a large increase (or decrease) in the risk of disease. (The stronger the association, the less likely it is to be due to bias or an unknown confounder.)

Dose-response relationship. Higher doses of the exposure are associated with higher rates of disease.

Biologic credibility. A plausible biologic mechanism is available to explain how the exposure causes disease.

Consistency. Other studies done in different ways and in different populations have found the same association.

Time sequence. The exposure can be shown to occur before the disease.

Specificity. The exposure is associated with a specific disease.

The above criteria are guidelines, not rules. Some toxicants that clearly cause disease do not meet all the above criteria. For example, cigarette smoking does not meet the specificity criterion, for it is associated with many diseases.

Cancer Clusters

When contamination is discovered in a community, citizens often look for health effects. They may notice a lot of people with cancer and conclude that this represents an unusually high incidence of disease. Public health agencies are often called upon to investigate the reported *cluster*—a group of individuals living in a limited area and manifesting a particular disease.

In many instances, scientists find that people have underestimated the background incidence of cancer and that the number of cancers is really just what would be expected.

In other situations, it is clear from the variety of cancers occurring that there is not a cluster that can be associated with a particular source. In the vast majority of cases, public health epidemiologists find that the suspected clusters do not represent unusual events.

Epidemiologists usually find that suspected clusters do not represent anything unusual.

4

Cancer Clusters (cont.)

Some cases are more complex than described on the previous page and it may not be possible to determine whether a cluster is present. Reasons why a firm conclusion is not possible include:

- the population is so small that any variations from population averages may be due to chance.

- it is usually impossible to reconstruct past exposures to the agent of concern to determine which cancer victims have been exposed and how much they have been exposed.

- the history of individual exposures to other possible cancer-causing agents, such as workplace chemicals or radon, cannot accurately be determined.

In summary, investigations of cancer clusters are very unlikely to establish a relationship between a local contaminant and the disease. However, public health epidemiologists often undertake cancer cluster analyses in response to strong public reaction to contamination incidents and deep public fear of cancer.

Conflicting Studies

What if researchers do not agree?
Reporters frequently are faced with
conflicting studies. (A recent example
is the question of whether alcohol
consumption increases the risk of breast
cancer; some studies say yes, some say
no.)

One possible explanation is that one
study was larger and therefore had
more power to find an effect. Other
possibilities are bias or confounding in
one or both studies. (See Chapter 5 for
discussion of how to evaluate the
validity of competing studies.)

Often, there is no obvious resolution to
the conflicts; they reflect the frustrating
fact that most diseases have complex,
intertwined causes that are difficult to
tease apart. The answers come slowly,
through the accumulation of research
results that eventually tip the balance in
favor of a particular explanation.

The answers to complex questions come slowly through the accumulation of study findings that eventually tip the balance in favor of a particular answer.

5 ASSESSING A STUDY'S VALIDITY

The perfect study has never been done, for there is always the possibility of human error in the study's design, execution, and analysis. How well a study is performed can be assessed to some degree by exploring how well the researchers sought to prevent and account for the common causes of distortion. These causes include chance, sample size, bias, and confounders.

Key Questions to Ask about a Study's Validity

(numbers indicate pages where more information can be found)

Chance

What is the probability that the study's results are due to chance? **63**

What is the study's 95% confidence interval [margin of error]?
65-68

Sample Size/Power

What was the sample size? How much power did the study have, with this sample size, to find an effect if one exists? **69-70**

Confounders

Are there confounders that could affect the study's results? What confounders did the investigators control for? **77-79**

Bias

   classification bias

How likely is it that people were misclassified? **71**

What did the investigators do to control misclassification?
71-73, 76

If one or two cases or controls were reclassified as exposed or unexposed, would the study's conclusions change?

   selection bias

How were the cases and controls in the study chosen? **75**

What are the possibilities for bias in the selection process?
74-75

What did the investigators do to try to prevent selection bias?
76

Other Studies

What have other investigators found? Are there other studies whose findings are similar to this study's findings? Are there studies that have different conclusions?

Factors Affecting Study Validity

The perfect study has never been done. Each study is performed at a distinct time and place with a unique group of subjects by investigators who utilize a particular study design. A diversity of methods are used to execute the study and to analyze its results. Chance always plays a part as well.

This is why different studies sometimes produce contradictory results. This is also why researchers almost never accept the results of a single study as definitive; the cumulative weight of evidence from several studies is necessary to draw sound conclusions.

How well a study is performed can be assessed to some degree by exploring how well the researchers sought to prevent and account for the common causes of distortion in a study.

In laboratory studies, the most common cause of distortion is chance, including the effects of sample size. For epidemiological studies, *bias* and *confounding*, as well as chance, are important factors to consider.

The results of a single study are seldom definitive because of the inevitable presence of chance and the possibility of improper study design.

5

Chance

All experimental and epidemiological studies are based on samples from larger populations. An epidemiological study that compares the incidence of lung cancer among smokers and nonsmokers, for example, uses a group of smokers selected from the population of all smokers, and a group of nonsmokers selected from the population of all nonsmokers.

The use of samples inevitably introduces uncertainty into the results. Any sample will, by chance, differ at least a little from its parent population. The smaller the sample and the more diverse the parent population, the more likely the sample will differ from the parent population.

In any study comparing two groups, at least some of the difference between groups is due to this sampling effect.

Scientists use mathematical tests, based on the science of statistics, to estimate the size of the sampling effect and, therefore, the amount of uncertainty associated with the study's findings. The results of these statistical tests are commonly expressed as *p values* and *confidence intervals* (see following pages).

Observed differences between groups of experimental animals or between populations of humans may be due to chance rather than due to real differences.

Example of chance: Assume two populations each have a 10% incidence of a particular disease. A random sample from one could, by chance, end up with 15% sick people and a sample from the other, 9% sick people. To an observer, it might appear that one population had a higher incidence of disease, while no difference actually existed.

Measures of Chance

P Values

A *p value* (probability value) shows the probability that the differences observed between two samples are due to chance variation in the samples rather than true differences in the parent populations.

P values range from 0 to 1. The closer the p value is to zero, the greater the likelihood that the difference between two samples reflects a real difference between the parent populations.

Although p values are not presented with percentage signs, you can think of them as representing a 0% to 100% probability that the observed difference is due to chance.

P values indicate the probability that observed differences are due to chance rather than reflecting true differences.

5

Example of p values: A p value of 0.001 (0.1%) means that only one time in a thousand would the difference observed be due to chance. A p value of 0.05 (5%) means that 5 times in 100 the observed difference would be due to chance. In other words, in the first example, there is a 99.9% probability that the difference is real. In the second example, there is a 95% probability that the difference is real.

A p value of 0.05 or smaller is usually the criteria used to indicate whether a study is statistically significant.

Measures of Chance (cont.)

P Values (cont.)

Traditionally, a p value of 0.05 (5%) or less is accepted as evidence that two populations are really different. A p value this small or smaller is taken to mean that the difference between the populations is *statistically significant.*

A p value of 0.05 represents a point on a continuum, not a scientific dividing line between "true" and "not true." A finding that has a p value of 0.06 (not statistically significant) could still reflect a true difference in the populations; a finding with a p value of 0.04 (statistically significant) could still be due to chance.

A scientist's conclusion that a difference between two samples reflects a true difference in the parent populations is as much a matter of judgment as of numbers.

Example of testing for chance using p values: In a clinical test of steroid injections for low back pain, doctors in Quebec City reported that 42% of 49 patients who received steroid injections experienced relief, compared to 33% of 48 patients who received injections of a harmless salt solution—a difference of 9%. Although it appears that steroids worked better than the placebo, a statistical test of the results yielded a p value of 0.50—that is, 50 times out of 100, samples of this size would be expected to show at least the observed 9% difference in pain relief, even if there were no difference in pain relief effectiveness between the steroids and the placebo. In other words, the results were not statistically significant, so this study offers no support for use of steroid injections in treating low back pain. It is still possible that steroids are effective in relieving pain, but that the sample size was too small to demonstrate the effect.

Measures of Chance (cont.)

Confidence Intervals

Estimates of risk based on limited data cannot perfectly reflect the real world; they almost certainly will be off by a little bit, and possibly by a great deal.

Pollsters acknowledge this uncertainty by providing margins of error for their polls. Laboratory scientists and epidemiologists call their margins of error *confidence intervals.*

When calculating risk ratios (see page 53), scientists have a process by which they use their data to calculate margins of error. Most of these margins of error are called 95% confidence intervals, meaning that there is a 95% probability that the risk will be no higher or lower than the extremes of this interval.

Confidence intervals provide a margin of error for the study's conclusions.

5

Example of testing for chance using confidence intervals: Chlorine in drinking water prevents epidemics of cholera and other water-borne illnesses, but a number of studies have suggested that chlorination also increases the risk of certain kinds of cancer. However, the studies' findings have been inconsistent, ranging from no risk of bladder cancer to a doubling of the risk. A group of researchers recently combined the results of 10 studies and reported that drinking chlorinated water is associated with a 38% increased risk of bladder cancer. But the 95% confidence interval was 1.01 to 1.87. In other words, the "best guess" is that the increased risk is 38%—but it could be as low as 1% or as high as 87%. And there is a 5% chance (five times out of 100) that a 95% confidence interval, does not include the true risk at all.

Measures of Chance (cont.)

Confidence Intervals (cont.)

Since a risk ratio of 1 means no additional risk of disease from the exposure (see page 54), a confidence interval that includes 1 (for example, 0.7-1.3) means that the data is not good enough to determine whether there is an increase, decrease, or no change in risk.

If, however, the confidence interval includes only numbers higher than 1 (for example, 1.1-1.5), a higher risk is likely. In this case, the risk is increased from 10% to 50%.

On the other hand, if the confidence interval is entirely below 1 (for example, 0.6-0.9), this suggests that the risk to the exposed population is only 60% to 90% of what it would have been without the exposure.

Confidence intervals below 1 indicate the suspect agent protects against disease; values near 1—it has no effect; over 1—it increases risk.

Example of confidence intervals: The chart below summarizes the results of several studies that examined the effect of vitamin B taken during pregnancy on the incidence of spinal cord defects in the baby. All of the studies showed a risk ratio below 1. However, the confidence interval in Study 1 ranged above 1, showing that the uncertainty in the study was too great to make a conclusion. In contrast, the confidence intervals of the other three studies included only values below 1, indicating vitamin B reduced the risk. Taking all the studies together, it can be concluded that vitamin B ingestion by pregnant women is likely to reduce the incidence of spinal cord defects in their offspring.

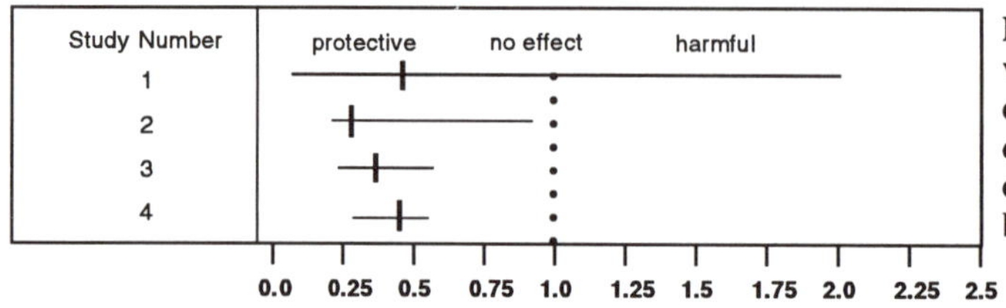

Effect of B vitamins taken during pregnancy on spinal cord defects in the baby.

Risk Ratio (vertical lines) With 95% Confidence Intervals (horizontal lines)

Measures of Chance (cont.)

Confidence Intervals in Epidemiological Studies

Confidence intervals are said to be wide if they contain a large range of values (e.g., 0.2 to 7.5), and narrow if they contain a small range of values (e.g., 2.5 to 3.0). The wider the interval, the less you can rely on the study.

In epidemiological studies, the width of the confidence interval is related to the sample size of the study. The larger the sample size, the narrower the confidence interval and the more precise the estimate of risk.

The width of the confidence interval is also related to the inherent variability of the factor being measured. The less the inherent variability, the narrower the confidence interval. (For example, body weight is highly variable, so a study of the effects of some factor on body weight would have a wider confidence interval than a similar study of the effects on head circumference, which is much less variable.)

P values and confidence intervals both are attempts to express the uncertainty associated with scientific studies. Most epidemiologists prefer confidence intervals because they provide more information than p values about the range of risk associated with an exposure.

Measures of Chance (cont.)

Confidence Intervals in Carcinogenesis Bioassays

In carcinogenesis bioassays, the results of administering a limited number of high doses to rodents are extrapolated downward to the lower doses that humans may encounter in the real environment. This process may cause considerable uncertainty about the risk at low doses. Confidence intervals describe the range of possible risk.

In practice, risk managers try to minimize the possibility of adverse impacts on human health. To build in a margin of safety, they generally report only the 95% upper confidence limit of the risk. This may erroneously give the impression that the 95% upper bound is the most likely estimate of the risk.

Example of using confidence intervals in carcinogenesis bioassays: There is concern about contaminants such as PCBs in fish, because they have been shown to cause cancer in laboratory animals. Risk managers wish to determine the risk of cancer for individuals who eat fish containing particular levels of PCBs. Extrapolating from laboratory animal studies, and calculating the 95% upper confidence limit, they may report that eating certain fish so many times a week will lead to an additional risk of cancer of 1 in 10,000. Because this risk number represents only the 95% upper confidence limit, it is likely that the true risk is much lower.

Sample Size

At least two possible explanations exist for results that indicate the substance under study has no effect on disease:

❏ there is no effect.

❏ there is an effect, but the study's sample size was too small to find it.

The probability of getting a statistically significant result—p less than or equal to 0.05—is closely tied to the size of the *sample* used in the study. The larger the sample size, the more information it contains, and the greater its ability to find an effect if one exists.

Small studies can reliably find only big risks.

Sample Size (cont.)

How large a sample is large enough? This depends on:

- ❏ how common the effect is.
- ❏ how much of an impact the suspected agent has on disease or effect rates.

The rarer the effect and/or the smaller the effect, the larger the sample needed to detect that effect. Small studies can reliably find only big risks.

A study's ability to find an effect is called its _power_. Formulas are available to calculate a study's power to find a specific-sized risk at different sample sizes. Typically, researchers would like a sample size large enough to have an 80% chance (80% power) of finding a doubling of the effect rate in the group exposed to the suspect agent.

(Ideally, researchers would like studies powerful enough to find any size risk. But such studies would be too expensive, take too long, and require too many participants to be feasible.)

Example of study size needed: Scientists believe that a high fat diet increases the risk of breast cancer. In order to have an 80% chance of detecting a 50% drop in breast cancer rates among women who halve their fat intake, researchers would need to enroll at least 30,000 women in a study and follow them for 10 years—and even then, there is a 20% chance (or 1 in 5) that the study would fail to detect the decline even if it occurred!

Bias and Confounders in Epidemiological Studies

Bias

An epidemiological study can be very large, very powerful—and very wrong.

Imbalances in the way researchers choose people for a study or systematic mistakes in the way they classify people as sick or well, exposed or unexposed, can produce a false relationship between an exposure and a disease. This distortion is called *bias*.

CLASSIFICATION ERRORS

Inevitably, some people in a study will be put in the wrong category of exposure or disease because of clerical errors, mistakes in the design or execution of the study, or an imperfect test for disease or exposure (no test is perfect). The question is: *was the study designed or conducted in a way likely to produce a lot of these mistakes?*

Even the findings from a powerful study can be wrong if researchers made mistakes in selecting or classifying subjects.

5

Bias and Confounders in Epidemiological Studies (cont.)

Bias (cont.)

CLASSIFICATION ERRORS (CONT.)

It is well-known that health status distorts memory of past events. People with disease are more likely to "remember" that they were exposed to a suspect substance whether they were or not; people who are healthy are more likely to forget past exposures. In a case-control study, this *recall bias* may produce a false association between an exposure and a disease.

People's recollections are influenced by whether they are sick and looking for a cause, or healthy and unconcerned.

Example of recall bias: Following widespread publicity about groundwater contamination in Santa Clara County, California, a case-control study found that women who recalled drinking tap water during their pregnancies had four times the risk of miscarriage as women who recalled drinking only bottled water. Later studies suggested that recall bias could account for much, if not all, of this association. Among other things:

❑ studies done after the publicity had died down found a smaller risk than studies done at the height of the publicity; and

❑ the association between tap water consumption and miscarriage was greater among women questioned by telephone interviewers (who knew whether they were talking to cases or controls) than among women who filled out mailed questionnaires.

Bias and Confounders in Epidemiological Studies (cont.)

Bias (cont.)

CLASSIFICATION ERRORS (CONT.)

If the study is not a blind study, problems may arise from investigators' and interviewers' unconscious desires to see what they want to see. Doctors who think an experimental drug is effective may be more likely to see improvement in patients taking the drug; interviewers who believe a chemical causes disease may question cases more closely than controls about possible exposures.

Sometimes, researchers will let their desire to see a certain result color their interpretation of the data.

Example of a classification error: In 1986, researchers at the University of California generated great excitement with a report from a clinical trial. They reported that patients with Alzheimer's disease who took the experimental drug Tacrine showed dramatic improvement in their mental function compared to Alzheimer's patients who took an inactive placebo. The report was considered especially promising because the study was supposedly *"double blind"*—neither researchers nor patients knew who was taking the real drug, so the researchers' evaluations of the patients' mental function could not be colored by their enthusiasm for the drug. A subsequent investigation by the Food and Drug Administration revealed that the researchers may indeed have known who was getting the real drug. In October 1992, a much larger, more rigorously controlled double blind study involving more than a dozen medical centers concluded that Tacrine did improve mental function, but so slightly that it was not noticeable to the evaluating doctors, and could be detected only by a battery of cognitive tests.

Bias (cont.)

SELECTION ERRORS

A military spokesman reported in 1992 that mail to the Joint Chiefs of Staff was running 4 to 1 against admitting gay people to the military. Most people would recognize that this mail survey may not represent the entire American public, because people who strongly opposed gays in the military were probably more moved to volunteer their opinions at that time, when the military was proposing to allow gays in the ranks, than were people who had other opinions or no opinion.

Selection bias occurs whenever the method of choosing participants results in a study group that differs from the parent population in ways that affect the study's conclusions. A major concern in epidemiological studies, selection bias can take many forms.

Selection bias, the tendency for study subjects to be different from the population, is a major concern in epidemiological studies.

Example of selection bias: Following publicity about fears of an increased risk of leukemia among soldiers who had been deliberately exposed to radiation during the Army's 1957 Smoky atomic bomb test, the federal Centers for Disease Control (CDC) conducted a study that did indeed find an association between leukemia and participation in Smoky. The CDC investigators tried to trace all the Smoky participants, but had better luck finding those who had developed cancer, since many of these ill soldiers contacted the CDC on their own initiative. This form of selection bias, called *volunteer bias*, could be responsible for the apparent association.

Bias and Confounders in Epidemiological Studies (cont.)

Bias—SELECTION ERRORS (CONT.)

To avoid selection bias, careful researchers take pains to assure that study subjects represent all who could have participated, and that comparison groups are selected the same way. But the selection method is seldom perfect. A major question in any epidemiological study is how much the results are skewed by selection bias.

Selection is seldom perfect, so the degree of selection bias is a relevant question to ask about any epidemiological study.

Examples of selection bias:

❐ A Virginia jazz enthusiast and medical school professor, attempting to refute the perception that jazz musicians live fast and die young, compared the average life expectancy in America with the age at death of 86 noted jazz musicians. He concluded that jazz musicians live longer. But his study's selection bias was immediately pointed out: people don't become jazz musicians until adulthood, after they have survived the perils of childhood. Since childhood deaths are critical in reducing average life expectancy, looking at average age at death is bound to show a survival advantage. A way to avoid this bias would be to look at age-specific mortality rates: for example, the mortality rate for 50-year-old jazz musicians compared to other 50-year-olds.

❐ National estimates of HIV infection rates in childbearing women were once based on screening of newborns' blood samples left over after other diagnostic tests were completed. But studies suggested that this practice seriously underestimated the true infection rate, because it tested only samples that contained sufficient leftover blood. Since HIV-infected newborns are sicker at birth, they undergo more tests, and their leftover samples often don't contain enough blood for screening. Therefore the blood that was screened was disproportionately from healthy babies. True HIV infection rates may be three times higher than these previous estimates.

All studies have some bias. The question is whether investigators took care to reduce bias as much as possible.

Bias and Confounders in Epidemiological Studies (cont.)

Bias (cont.)

PREVENTING BIAS

A good study will foresee and try to control bias. Researchers might:

- ❒ **Use memory aids** to avoid recall bias.

- ❒ **Lessen the chance of interviewers' influencing the responses** by not revealing to interviewers the study's exact purpose or whether the people they're interviewing are cases or controls.

- ❒ **Minimize dropouts** by recruiting participants for cohort studies from groups that are likely to be cooperative and easy to trace. Doctors and nurses are favored subjects for follow-up studies because they tend to be interested in research and are easy to trace through professional associations.

- ❒ **Choose more than one control group** for a case-control study. For example, if the study gets the same results with a control group selected from the cases' friends and a control group selected from the cases' work associates, it provides some assurance that the findings are real and not just artifacts of the control selection process.

All studies have some bias. The question is whether investigators took care to reduce bias as much as possible, and whether the findings could be easily explained by bias.

Bias and Confounders in Epidemiological Studies (cont.)

Confounding

Every morning at 10:00 a woman walks to the bus stop. At 10:01, a bus drives up and the woman gets on. A naive observer might conclude that the woman was responsible for the bus's arrival. In fact, both the woman's and the bus driver's behavior are driven by a hidden, third factor: the bus schedule.

The bus schedule is a confounder, producing an apparent cause-effect relationship between the woman's arrival and the bus's appearance.

Confounders are common in the study of disease. Confounders can:

❑ produce a spurious association between a harmless agent and a disease.

❑ mask an exposure's harmful effect.

Confounding occurs when a characteristic not considered by the researchers is in fact associated with both the disease and the suspected disease-causing agent.

Confounders are unmeasured characteristics that affect the study's outcome.

Example of a confounder: In the 1970s, a group opposed to fluoridation of water in the U.S. reported a dramatic increase in cancer death rates in 10 U.S. cities that had switched to fluoridated water. But other investigators noted that the populations of these cities had changed dramatically in the same period, with growing proportions of elderly people and black people—groups at higher risk of cancer. After taking into account the confounding effects of age and race, the investigators found that these cities' cancer death rates actually had dropped since the introduction of fluoridated water.

Bias and Confounders in Epidemiological Studies (cont.)

Confounding (cont.)

Age, sex, race, income, and cigarette smoking are among the most common confounders, because they affect the risk of many diseases and also are closely linked with other exposures that might be investigated as causes of disease. If a researcher does not at least take these factors into account when looking at causes of disease, the study is suspect.

Age, race, sex, income, and cigarette smoking are common confounders.

Example of confounders:

❑ Early epidemiological studies noted that the more children a woman had, the lower her risk of breast cancer. However, investigators quickly realized that a woman with a large family tends to be relatively young at the birth of her first child. Subsequent studies showed that it was young age at first birth, not number of full-term pregnancies, that reduces breast cancer risk. The apparent association between large families and lower breast cancer risk was the result of the confounding effect of age at first birth. (Note that older age at first birth does not directly "cause" breast cancer; it is probably a proxy for hormonal changes related to pregnancy.)

❑ A difficulty in investigating occupational hazards is the problem of disentangling the effects of work place chemicals from the effects of lifestyle choices, like smoking habits. Chemicals in the work place are suspected causes of lung and bladder cancers. Smoking also causes these diseases. Blue collar workers are both more likely to smoke and more likely to have jobs that expose them to chemicals. A study that found an association between a work place chemical and lung cancer would be inconclusive unless it could rule out smoking as a possible confounder of the reported association.

Bias and Confounders in Epidemiological Studies (cont.)

Confounding (cont.)

Epidemiologists use a number of techniques to try to remove the distorting effect of confounders. They can restrict study subjects to one age group, sex, or race. Or they can use statistical techniques that show the effect on disease of the agent of interest with all known confounding factors held constant. The problem with these techniques is that they can control only for confounders the investigators have identified. A major concern is whether the investigators have overlooked a confounder and have not controlled for it.

A major concern is whether researchers have overlooked a confounder and therefore have not controlled for it.

5

6 RISK COMMUNICATION BASICS

Audience reactions to risk information are sometimes surprising. Citizen reaction to risk messages is coming under increasing study by communication, psychology, and social science experts. Their findings are helping reporters to formulate stories that increase public understanding.

Acknowledgments

Much of the information in this chapter was drawn from the research of several individuals on the cutting edge of risk perception and risk communication research. Chief among them are: Vincent Covello, Columbia University, New York, New York; Michael R. Edelstein, Ramapo College of New Jersey, Mahwah, New Jersey; Baruch Fishoff, Carnegie Mellon University, Pittsburgh, Pennsylvania; Peter Sandman, Rutgers University, New Brunswick, New Jersey; Paul Slovic, Decision Research, Inc., Eugene, Oregon. See Recommended Reading for a listing of publications and articles by these researchers and others.

Key Risk Communication Points to Remember

(numbers indicate pages where more information can be found)

Emotional reactions to risk news—called "outrage"—play a bigger role in public reaction than the scientific information. **84-86**

Outrage is based on psychologically valid factors and is not illogical. **87-88**

Reporters can address outrage by providing information that increases the audience's understanding of the hazard and shows them how to gain some control of the situation. **89-90**

Risk comparisons and analogies should be done in the spirit of increasing the audience's understanding, not to minimize (or maximize) the risk they face. **91-92**

Outrage tends to focus on sudden, involuntary risks, while ongoing hazards like radon or self-imposed lifestyle risks are ignored or minimized. **83-84, 94**

Introduction

A hazardous waste management company plans to locate a new incinerator in your community. Residents are fearful of future emissions; officials declare there is nothing to worry about. A drawn-out controversy is expected. What features of citizen reaction to potential risk should you know so you can present the information in a way that helps people respond constructively?

As a reporter, you may do all you can to understand risk issues and report them clearly. Yet your audience's reactions may not be what you had expected. For example, they may not take serious hazards—like radon or high-fat diets—seriously, yet they may remain agitated about relatively insignificant hazards—like pesticide residues in food or nuclear power generation.* What's going on?

Citizen reaction to risk messages is a fascinating field coming under increasing study by communication, psychology, and social science experts. Their findings provide insights that will help you formulate your stories so they increase public understanding.

Researchers are uncovering the reasons that citizen reaction to risk news is sometimes the opposite of what is expected.

6

---

* Health officials rate chemicals in food as trivial risks, but view high-fat diets as important causes of cancer. Likewise, health problems from nuclear power plant radiation cannot compare with the estimated 5,000-20,000 cancer deaths/year from radon.

Outrage

The hazard of radon—the number of people killed—is much greater than the hazard of nuclear power. Yet Americans are much more up in arms about nuclear power. Why is this?

Risk communication experts point to a factor they call "outrage." Outrage* refers to the level of public anger and fear about an environmental risk issue. Outrage has a much greater influence on citizens' reactions to a hazard than the scientifically calculated risk.

When people become outraged, they may overreact. Conversely, if people are not outraged, they may underreact.

Emotional responses to risk news—called "outrage"—play a bigger role in public reaction than the scientific information.

---

* The term "outrage" was coined by Dr. Peter Sandman, Professor of Environmental Journalism and Director of the Environmental Communication Research Program, Rutgers University. It is based on the research of a number of leading psychologists and risk perception experts.

Outrage (cont.)

Outrage Factors

What causes outrage? People become outraged—fearful, angry, frustrated—if the risk is perceived to be:

involuntary: People don't like to be forced to face a risk—like trace chemicals in tap water. (But they will voluntarily assume risks—like drinking diet soda.)

uncontrollable: When preventing risk is in someone else's hands (government or industry), citizens feel helpless to change the situation. If the citizen can prevent or reduce the risk (using household chemicals properly) the risk is more acceptable.

immoral: Pollution is viewed as an evil. Therefore, people consider it unethical for governments and industries to claim that a risk is acceptable based on cost-benefit analysis or because there is "only" a low incidence of harm.

unfamiliar: An industrial process producing an unpronounceable chemical is a much less acceptable risk than something more everyday, like driving a car or eating junk food.

dreadful: A risk that could cause a much-feared or dread disease (like most cancers) is seen as more dangerous than a risk that could cause a less-feared disease.

uncertain: People become uneasy when scientists are not certain about the risk posed by a hazard—its exact effect, severity, or prevalence.

Outrage factors are those components of a risk situation that cause fear, anger, defensiveness, or frustration.

6

Outrage (cont.)

Outrage Factors (cont.)

catastrophic: A risk resulting in a large-scale disastrous event (plane crash, nuclear reactor meltdown), is more dreaded than a risk affecting individuals singly (auto accidents, radon).

memorable: A potential risk similar to a remarkable event imbedded in the memory, like Bhopal or Three Mile Island, is viewed as much more dangerous than the risk of some unheard-of or little-known disease.

unfair: People become outraged if they feel they are being wrongfully exposed. For example:

❑ exposure to a risk that people in a neighboring community or a different economic bracket are not being exposed to.

❑ exposure to a risk with no benefit, e.g., living next to a nuclear waste dump, but receiving no benefit from nuclear power generation. In contrast, people will assume the risk of exposure to something like medical X-rays because they perceive a benefit that equals or outweighs the risk.

untrustworthy: People become outraged if they have no confidence in the source of the risk, such as industry or government. In contrast they will accept risks from what they view as a reliable risk source, such as a doctor.

Emotional Reactions Valid

Clearly, emotions play a large role in public perception of risk. No explanation of scientific findings makes much impression if people are either hysterical or agitated.

This emotional response is viewed by many with technical training as irrational, and they therefore ignore it or condemn it.

In fact, individual emotional responses are based on psychologically valid factors and are, from the psychological perspective, perfectly rational. When people become aware of a threat, they are naturally inclined to:

☐ fear the unknown.

☐ want to maintain control.

☐ protect home and family.

☐ be alienated by dependence on others (government, industry officials).

☐ protect their belief in a just world.

Outrage is based on valid psychological needs that must be recognized and met before a mutually acceptable solution can be found.

6

Emotional Reactions Valid (cont.)

By contrast, technically trained officials tend to trust scientific analyses, accept the effectiveness of engineering solutions and contingency plans, and to believe that experts know best.

Thus, much of the conflict surrounding risk issues is a result of groups with vastly different values becoming pitted against one another.

Communications experts urge those involved in communicating risk—officials and reporters—to accept the reality and validity of the public's emotions, and to seek ways of communicating that take these emotions into account.

Officials rely on a technically based value system that does not recognize the basis of outrage. Thus conflict arises between officials and citizens in risk situations.

Risk Communication Guidelines

Here are some ways that reporters (and officials) can address the psychological factors influencing citizen response to hazards. The point, of course, is not to diminish legitimate concerns, or heighten illegitimate ones, but to encourage constructive action.

❏ Describe what individuals can do to reduce their exposure.

❏ Describe what industry and government are/are not doing to reduce the risk.

❏ Describe the benefits as well as the risks to the specific audience (not just society in general) of the substance/process of concern.

❏ Describe the alternatives and their risks.

❏ Describe what people can do to get involved in the decisionmaking process.

❏ Provide information that will help the audience to evaluate the risk (see next page).

Reporters can provide information that helps their audience understand and control the risk.

Reporters can provide their audiences with information that will help them evaluate the risk information they see or hear.

Helping the Audience Evaluate Risk

Ultimately, citizens judge how dangerous a risk is and whether they should take action to reduce it. Reporters can play a key role in encouraging sound decisions by providing information that will help their audience evaluate the risk. Some fundamental information is:

❑ How much of the substance is the audience actually being exposed to?

❑ What is the likelihood of accidental exposure? What safety/back-up measures are in place?

❑ What is the legal standard for the substance? Is the standard controversial or widely accepted as sound?

❑ What health or environmental problems is the standard based on? Are there other problems that should be considered?

❑ Is the source of the risk information reputable? Who funded the work? What do other sources say?

❑ Were the studies done on a population similar to this audience?

❑ What are the benefits of the substance/facility? What are the trade-offs?

❑ How does the risk compare with other risks this audience faces? (See next page.)

Risk Comparisons

Risk comparisons—comparing a new, unfamiliar risk with an old, familiar one—are appealing because they provide a concrete way to express a numerical concept (such as one death in a million). Risk comparisons appear to establish a scale of severity by which people can judge whether the new risk is something to be concerned about.

However, risk comparisons must be used with great care. Often, an involuntary risk is compared with a voluntary one (e.g., the risk from nearby chemical plant emissions is compared with smoking, dietary habits, or some other lifestyle choice). Such comparing of an involuntary exposure to risk with a voluntary exposure tends not to influence people's perceptions.

If such a comparison is done in the spirit of minimizing the importance of the involuntary risk, it will generate anger.

The value of risk comparisons is also limited by the fact that risks tend to accumulate in people's minds. No matter how small the new risk, people are inclined to see it as simply one more unwelcome vexation to add to their already heavy burden of coping with modern-day problems.

Risk comparisons that contrast an involuntary risk with a voluntary one typically generate anger rather than understanding.

6

Risk Comparisons (cont.)

Several types of risk comparisons are generally more useful than comparing involuntary risks with voluntary ones. These are:

❏ comparisons of similar risks.
❏ comparisons of risks with benefits.
❏ comparisons of alternative substances/methods.
❏ comparisons to natural background levels.
❏ comparisons with a regulatory standard.

The most useful risk comparisons compare similar risks, compare risks with alternatives, or compare risks with benefits.

Examples of risk comparisons:

❏ **Comparisons of similar risks:** How do synthetic pesticide levels in a food compare with the levels of natural pesticides found in many foods?

❏ **Comparisons of risks with benefits:** The risk to human health of using chlorine to disinfect drinking water vs. chlorine's role in protecting human life from infectious diseases.

❏ **Comparisons of alternatives:** Incineration of a waste versus landfilling it—which actually causes the most pollution of the environment?

❏ **Comparisons to natural background levels:** How does the level of a substance in a suspected contaminated area compare with natural background levels—such as the level of lead in someone's backyard compared with the average natural lead levels in soils in the United States.

❏ **Comparisons with a regulatory standard:** How does the comparison of arsenic in a city's drinking water compare with the standard set by the Environmental Protection Agency?

Concentration Analogies

Explaining chemical concentrations (parts per million, parts per billion) by using analogies (1 ppm = 1 drop of gas in an auto gas tank) appeals to the imagination and helps people understand the magnitude of a concentration.

Like risk comparisons, however, analogies can cause anger if used merely to minimize the magnitude, and thus the risk.

Analogies should be accompanied by information on the significance of the concentration—its effect on human health, the environment, etc.

See Appendix 1 for a sampling of concentration analogies.

Covering Chronic Risks

Many risk communication experts assert that people's tendency to overestimate sudden, imposed risk and underestimate chronic or lifestyle-imposed risks is reinforced by generally more extensive media coverage of accidents and disasters than of chronic situations.

These experts encourage reporters to be persistent in their coverage of the chronic risks—those due to diet, lifestyle, or home contaminants such as radon, lead, and asbestos.

Researchers are studying how to present risk messages about chronic or lifestyle risks in a manner that results in the individual taking corrective action. Findings to date are tentative.*

---

* For the latest information, contact the Environmental Communication Research Program, Cook College, Rutgers University, P.O. Box 231, New Brunswick, NJ 08903.

APPENDICES

GLOSSARY

RECOMMENDED READING

INDEX   111

APPENDIX 1: CONCENTRATION ANALOGIES

One Part Per Million

- one automobile in bumper-to-bumper traffic from Cleveland to San Francisco
- one pancake in a stack four miles high
- 1 inch in 16 miles
- one minute in two years
- one ounce in 32 tons
- one cent in $10,000
- .0001% (or 10,000 ppm equals 1%)

One Part Per Billion

- one 4-inch hamburger in a chain of hamburgers circling the earth at the equator two-and-a-half times
- one silver dollar in a roll of silver dollars stretching from Detroit to Salt Lake City
- one bogie in 3,500 golf tournaments
- one kernel of corn in a 45-foot high, 16-foot diameter silo
- one sheet in a roll of toilet paper stretching from New York to London
- one second of time in 32 years

One Part Per Trillion

- one square foot of floor tile on a kitchen floor the size of Indiana
- one drop of detergent in enough dishwater to fill a string of railroad tank cars ten miles long
- one square inch in 250 square miles
- one mile on a 2-month journey at the speed of light

One Part Per Quadrillion

- one postage stamp on a letter the size of California and Oregon
- one human hair out of all the hair on all the heads of all the people in the world
- one mile on a journey of 170 light years

APPENDIX 2: INFORMATION SOURCES

Listed here are a few key toll-free hotline information sources on topics related to environmental health risks. Check the Recommended Reading list for publications with more extensive lists of information sources. In particular, Sachsman et al., *Environmental Reporter's Handbook,* and Ward, *Chemicals, the Press, and the Public,* provide extensive lists of information sources.

Cancer Issues
National Cancer Institute, Cancer Information Service
1-800-4-CANCER

Chemical Emergencies
Chemical Manufacturers Association
1-800-424-9300

Chemical Names and Manufacturers
Chemical Manufacturers Association
1-800-262-8200

Environmental Health Issues
U.S. EPA, Public Information Center
1-800-828-4445

Hazardous Waste Sites
Enviro-Health Clearinghouse
1-800-643-4794

Pesticides
National Pesticide Telecommunications Network
1-800-858-7378

Physicians
American College of Physicians
1-800-523-1546

Scientific Experts

Scientists' Institute for Public Information (SIPI)
Media Resource Service
1-800-223-1730
In New York, call 1-212-661-9110

This service for journalists will provide names and numbers of many of the nation's most qualified experts on chemical substances. Will refer you to specialists with different viewpoints.

Spills

National Response Center, Oil and Chemical Spill Hotline
1-800-424-8802

Toxic Substances

Natural Resources Defense Council
1-800-424-9065

Worker Exposure

Enviro-Health Clearinghouse
1-800-643-4794

GLOSSARY

Numbers indicate pages in the text where the term can be found. Italicized words in the definitions are also defined in this Glossary.

Toxicological, Epidemiological, and Chemical Terms

adsorption: Uptake of water or dissolved chemicals by a cell or an organism. Movement of a chemical into or across a tissue. **23**

accumulation: Buildup of a chemical in the body due to long-term or repeated exposure.

acute toxicity: Causing adverse effects that occur very rapidly after a single exposure has occurred. **30, 32, 33**

action level: A concentration of a specific substance that when exceeded, triggers risk management activities designed to protect human health.

additive effect: Combined effect of two or more chemicals equal to the sum of their individual effects.

aerosol: A mixture of very small particles of a liquid or a solid in a gas.

antagonism: Combined action of two or more substances to produce an effect less than the sum of their individual effects; the opposite of synergism.

antidote: A therapeutic agent administered to counteract the effect of a toxic agent.

association: A relationship between an exposure and a disease. The relationship does not of itself confirm that the exposure caused the disease. **44, 54, 72, 77, 101**

bias: A distortion of the facts caused by errors in selecting or classifying the subjects of a study. **60, 61, 71-79, 106, 107**

bioassay: A technique for evaluating the biological activity or potency of a substance by testing its effect on an organism. **31, 34, 38-41, 68**

carcinogen: Any substance capable of producing or inducing cancer.

carcinogenesis bioassay: A method of testing a substance for carcinogenic effects that utilizes high-dose studies on laboratory animals to look for even the rare case of cancer. **31, 34, 38-41, 68**

case-control study: Epidemiological method used to search for the cause(s) of disease. Researchers assemble a group of people with disease (cases) and a group without disease (controls) and look for differences that could explain why one group is sick and the other is not. **48, 50, 76**

chronic toxicity: Causing adverse effects that occur after repeated exposures over a long period of time. **30, 31, 34**

clinical trial: An experiment to examine the effect of a treatment on disease. Patients with disease are randomly assigned to receive the treatment or an inert placebo (or a different treatment), and are followed to determine which group does better. **51, 52**

cluster: A group of individuals living in a limited area and manifesting a particular disease. **55, 56**

cohort study: Epidemiological method used to search for the cause(s) of disease. Groups of people whose members differ on one or more characteristic(s) suspected of causing disease are followed over time to see if the people with the characteristic(s) get more disease. **48-50, 76**

comparison study: A study that involves comparison of two or more groups. See *case control study, cohort study, cross-sectional study,* and *clinical trial.*

confidence interval: The margin of error calculated for a risk estimate. 95% confidence intervals are the most common, meaning that there is a 95% probability that the risk is no higher or lower than the range of values included in this interval. **62, 65-68**

confounder: A cause of disease that is not under investigation, but that distorts the cause-effect relationship under study. **77-79**

control group: A group of experimental subjects not exposed to a substance or treatment being investigated and compared to experimental groups that are exposed. **48, 73, 76**

cross-sectional study: Epidemiological method used to determine whether a problem exists that warrants further study. A population of interest is identified and the individuals asked about current illnesses and current exposures. **51**

dose: a measure of exposure. Dose is often expressed in milligrams per kilogram (mg/kg) or parts per million (ppm).

dose-response study: A study in which the amount of substance (dose) is gradually increased and the effects at each dose are noted. Performed on animals, commonly mice or rats. Used to determine both acute and chronic non-carcinogenic toxicity. **31, 35, 36, 38**

double-blind: A type of clinical trial in which neither the patients nor the researchers responsible for observing the effects and analyzing the data know who is getting the treatment and who is getting an inactive placebo until the experiment ends. **73**

environmental exposure study: Estimates how much of a substance is/was present in the environment and how much people come into contact with. Used to assess long-term exposures. **17, 19, 21-24**

epidemiology: The study of patterns of disease in populations. Crucial to the study of links between environmental agents and human diseases. **45**

exposure: (1) The amount, frequency, and duration of contact with an environmental agent. (2) In epidemiology, anything that increases the likelihood of disease. See *risk factor*. **47**

exposure assessment: A step in risk assessment that estimates how much of a substance people are actually exposed to. **4, 6, 14-26**

extrapolate: Estimate or infer something by extending or projecting known information. For example, the future incidence of AIDS can be extrapolated from its current prevalence and trends. **7**

follow-up study: A *cohort study*. **49**

hazardous: The potential that the use of a product will result in an adverse effect on humans or the environment in a given situation. The degree of hazard is based on the substance's characteristics, such as toxicity, flammability, explosiveness, corrosiveness, etc., and the ease with which people or the environment can come in contact with it. Hazardous is not the same as *toxicity*, which refers exclusively to systemic damage to a living organism. **29**

hazardous: A general term to denote any substance that is either a physical hazard (such as an explosive) or a health hazard (such as a poison or carcinogen). *Toxic* is a more specific term referring only to health hazards. **29**

in vitro: Literally, "in glass." Usually refers to a laboratory test. **5**

in vivo: Refers to a study of chemical effects conducted in intact living organisms.

LC$_{50}$: The concentration in the air that will kill half of the test animals—in other words the lethal concentration for 50% of the animals. Exposure is usually from one to four hours. The value is expressed in mg/liter, mg/m^3, or ppm. Also written as LC-50. **32**

LD$_{50}$: The quantity of material that when ingested, injected, or applied to the skin in a single dose will kill half of the test animals in 14 days—in other words the lethal dose for 50% of the animals. The value is expressed in g/kg or mg/kg of body weight. The test animal and test conditions should be specified. Also written as LD-50. **32, 33**

LD$_{50}$ study, LC$_{50}$ study: A type of dose-response study used to determine the acute toxicity of a substance. Performed on animals, the results are *extrapolated* to assess acute toxicity in humans. **32**

lethal amount: A measure of acute toxicity calculated by multiplying the *LD$_{50}$* by a number representing average human weight. **33**

LOAEL (lowest observable adverse effect level): In a dose-response study, the smallest dose that causes any detectable *adverse* effect. **35**

LOEL (lowest observable effect level): In a dose-response study, the smallest dose that causes any detectable effect. **35**

mathematical model: A set of equations that attempt to mimic a real situation and predict what will happen under different circumstances. **23, 39-42**

NOAEL (no observable adverse effect level): In a dose-response study, the highest dose at which no observable *adverse* effects occur. **36**

NOEL (no observable effect level): In a dose-response study, the highest dose at which no observable effects occur. **36**

odds ratio: See definition for *risk ratio.*

organic chemicals: Strictly speaking, these are chemical compounds that include carbon, although simple carbon compounds such as carbon dioxide (CO$_2$) are not usually referred to as organic. In common usage, organic chemicals are hydrocarbons—those carbon compounds consisting of a carbon chain or ring with hydrogen attached along with a variety of other elements. DDT, PCBs, dioxin, and many other pesticides and synthetic industrial chemicals are organic chemicals.

personal exposure study: Calculates how much of a substance people are exposed to by analyzing bodily fluids or tissue. **17, 19, 20**

pH: A measure of relative acidity and alkalinity. A pH of 7 indicates a neutral substance; higher values indicate increasing alkalinity; lower values indicate increasing acidity.

poison: A substance or mixture that can cause death or serious harm; usually refers to acute effects.

population: Any group about which a researcher wants to draw conclusions based on a sample. Elementary school students in Detroit, people in the U.S. who smoke marijuana, and employees of a state Department of Public Health are examples of populations. **45, 56, 62, 74**

power: A study's ability to find an effect, expressed as a percent from 0 to 100. The larger the sample size, the more likely it is that the study will find an effect, if one exists. **70**

prospective study: A *cohort study.*

p value (probability value): A measure of chance. Measures the probability that a study's results are due to chance variations in the samples and do not reflect a true difference in the populations. P values range from 0.0 to 1. The closer the p value is to zero, the more likely the study results are real. A p value of 0.05 or less is usually accepted as evidence that the difference observed is not due to chance, but reflects a true difference between the populations. **62-64, 67, 69**

recall bias: A tendency for people experiencing toxic effects to be more likely to remember exposures than people who have not been affected. **72**

relative risk: See definition for *risk ratio.*

risk assessment: As used in this handbook, a scientific process that estimates the type and magnitude of risk to human health posed by exposure to chemical substances. **2-14**

risk characterization: The final step in risk assessment. Combines information on toxicity and exposure to describe what the risk is likely to be. **4, 8** *risk factor:* In epidemiology, anything that increases the likelihood of disease. Also called *exposure.* **47**

risk management: The effort to reduce or manage risk through education, regulation, and clean-up. Risk managers use the results of risk assessments, plus economic, social, and legal considerations to make regulatory and policy decisions. **12, 36**

risk ratio: A number that indicates how much more or less likely people with a suspect characteristic are to show the effects in question (such as, how much more likely are people who smoke to die of lung cancer than people who don't smoke). It is calculated by dividing the proportion of people who are affected (die of lung cancer) and have the suspect characteristic (smoke) by the proportion of people who are affected (die of lung cancer) and do not have the suspect characteristic (do not smoke). **53**

safety factor: A number (equal to or great than one) divided into *NOAEL* or *LOAEL* values derived from measurements in animals or small groups of humans, in order to estimate a NOAEL or LOAEL value for the whole human population. **12, 28, 36, 37**

sample: A group of people selected from a population and studied in order to draw conclusions about the entire population. **62, 69, 70**

selection bias: A tendency for study subjects to differ from the population they are supposed to represent in a way that affects their risk of adverse effects. **74, 75**

statistically significant: The value researchers select as a basis for accepting the results of a study as "true," that is, unlikely to be due to chance. Traditionally, researchers have selected a *p value* of 0.05 as the cutoff; results with p values at or below 0.05 are deemed statistically significant. **64, 69**

teratogen: A substance that can cause malformation in the fetus following exposure of the mother.

threshold: The lowest dose of a chemical at which a specific effect is observed and below which it is not observed. **31, 41**

toxicity: The inherent potential of a substance to cause systemic damage to living organisms. **29**

toxic substance: A substance that can cause acute or chronic adverse effects on living organisms.

toxicity assessment: The step in risk assessment that looks at how much of a substance causes what kind of harm. **4, 7, 28-41**

volunteer bias: A type of selection bias in which the study group includes people who volunteered for the study instead of being selected by some random process. Volunteers tend to differ in important ways from the population they are supposed to represent, and these differences often affect the risk of toxic effects. **74**

<: less than. Read $p < 0.5$ as p is less than 0.5.

>: greater than. Read $p > 0.5$ as p is greater than 0.5.

Units of Measure

FOR SOLIDS

g: gram; a metric unit of weight; there are one thousand grams in a kilogram.

g/kg: grams per kilogram.

kg: kilogram; a metric unit of weight equalling approximately 2.2 U.S. pounds.

mg: milligram; a metric unit of weight; there are one thousand milligrams in a gram.

mg/kg: milligrams per kilogram. Often used to express a toxicological dose.

FOR LIQUIDS

cc: cubic centimeter; similar to a milliliter.

L: liter; a metric unit of volume or capacity. A U.S. quart is about 9/10 of a liter.

ml: milliliter; a metric unit of volume or capacity; there are one thousand milliliters in a liter. One milliliter equals one cubic centimeter.

FOR GASES

mg/m³: milligrams per cubic meter of air.

mg/l: milligrams per liter of air.

GENERAL

ppb: parts per billion. See Appendix 1 for useful analogies.

ppm: parts per million. See Appendix 1 for useful analogies.

RECOMMENDED READING

Chemicals, the Press, and the Public: A Journalist's Guide to Reporting on Chemicals in the Community.
Ward, Bud.
Washington, D.C.: Environmental Health Center, National Safety Council. 122 pp.

Explains how journalists can "access" information on chemicals now available under the Federal Emergency Planning and Community Right-to-Know Act of 1986. Describes how a reporter should cover an emergency (chemical spill) and provides a checklist of questions to ask. Includes long list of state and federal information sources.

Environmental Reporter's Handbook.
Sachsman, David B., Michael R. Greenberg, and Peter M. Sandman. 1988.
Newark: New Jersey Institute of Technology. 175 pp.
(Contact: Environmental Communication Research Program, Cook College, Rutgers University, 122 Ryders Lane, New Brunswick, NJ 08903)

Contains 2-4 page briefings on the most common types of environmental news stories from acid rain to pesticides to landfills. The briefings present an overview of the issue, sources of information for the reporter, and pitfalls for the reporter to avoid. Also includes a large directory of information sources, bibliography, glossary, and list of acronyms.

Epidemiology for Journalists.
Wartenberg, Daniel.
Los Angeles: Foundation for American Communications. 41 pp.

Explains the principles of epidemiology in a clearly written style, with good use of illustrative examples. Covers the types of epidemiological studies, the problems encountered in these studies, and a guide to statistics and data analysis. Key questions to ask epidemiologists and a glossary are also included. A quick read with lots of information.

Health Risks and the Press.
Moore, Mike (ed.). 1989.
Washington, D.C.: The Media Institute. 112 pp.

Focuses on the relationship between reporters and scientists.
Includes a few tips for reporters. Separate essays. Includes illustrative examples, broader perspectives.

News and Numbers: A Guide to Reporting Statistical Claims and Controversies in Health and Other Fields.
Cohn, Victor. 1989.
Ames: Iowa State University Press. 180 pp.

Explains statistics as they relate to a wide range of issues, including environmental risks, health, politics, and economics. Gives questions reporters can ask and explains their significance.
No-nonsense, readable treatment of the meaning of scientists' numbers.

Reporting on Risk: Getting it Right in an Age of Risk.
Cohn, Victor. 1990.
Washington, D.C.: The Media Institute. 65 pp.

Discusses need for better reporting and reasons why it is difficult.
Explains some basic rules of science, statistics, and toxicology.
Lists questions reporters should ask. Includes bibliography.

Toxic Substances and Risk

A Primer on Toxicology Principles and Applications.
Kamrin, Michael. 1988.
Chelsea, MI: Lewis Publishers.

Presents basic toxicology principles in a sophisticated yet nontechnical style. Provides an understanding of both the strengths and limitations of the discipline of toxicology.

Breaking the Vicious Circle.
Breyer, S. 1993.
Cambridge, MA: Harvard University Press.

Presents a critical analysis of the current way that environmental risks are assessed and managed in the U.S. and suggests a method of improving the current situation to more effectively and efficiently reduce risk.

Phantom Risks: Scientific Inference and the Law.
Foster, K.R., D.E. Bernstein, and P.W. Huber (eds.). 1993.
Cambridge, MA: MIT Press.

Evaluates health risks from environmental hazards, especially those
that have been the subject of litigation. Explores the contrast
between the ease with which a substance becomes suspect and the
difficulty of actually proving a connection between the substance
and health.

The Book of Risks.
Laudan, Larry. 1994.
New York: Wiley & Sons.

Lists the statistical odds associated with many risks, both common
and obscure.

**The Dose Makes the Poison: A Plain-Language Guide
to Toxicology.**
Ottoboni, M. Alice. 1991.
New York: Van Nostrand Reinhold.

A clearly written primer on toxicity, risk assessment, and epidemiology. Glossary and index enhance usefulness.

Toxic Terror: The Truth Behind the Cancer Scares.
Whelan, E. M. 1993.
Buffalo, NY: Prometheus Books.

Evaluates the risks presented by asbestos, dioxin, nuclear power,
pesticides, and PCBs.

**Up to Your Armpits in Alligators? How to Sort Out What Risks
are Worth Worrying About!**
Paling, John and Sean Paling. 1993.
Gainesville, FL: The Environmental Institute.
(Contact: The Environmental Institute, 5822 N.W. 91st Blvd.,
Gainesville, FL 32653)

Presents an "environmental Richter scale" by which to rank and
compare risks.

Publications on Risk Communication

BOOKS

Contaminated Communities: The Social and Psychological Impacts of Residential Toxic Exposure.
Edelstein, Michael R. 1988.
Westview Publishers.

Environmental Risk and the Press: An Exploratory Assessment.
Sandman, Peter M., David B. Sachsman, Michael R. Greenberg, and Michael Gochfeld. 1987.
New Brunswick, NJ: Transaction Books.

Reporting on Risk: How the Mass Media Portray Accidents, Diseases, Disasters, and Other Hazards.
Singer, Eleanor and Phyllis M. Endreny. 1993.
New York: Russel Sage Foundation.

Tainted Truth: The Manipulation of Fact in America.
Crossen, Cynthia. 1994.
New York: Simon and Schuster.

What are the Chances? Risks, Odds, and Likelihood in Everyday Life.
Siskin, Bernard, Jerome Staller, and David Rorvik. 1990.
New York: A Plume Book.

JOURNAL AND MAGAZINE ARTICLES

Communicating Right-to-Know Information on Chemical Risks.
Covello, Vincent T. 1989.
Environmental Science and Technology 23:1444-1449.

Explaining Risk to Non-Experts.
Sandman, Peter M. 1987.
Emergency Preparedness Digest. Oct.-Dec., pp. 25-29.

Informing and Educating the Public About Risk.
Slovic, P. 1986.
Risk Analysis 4:403-415.

Media Coverage of a Crisis: Better Than Reported, Worse Than Necessary.
Scanlon, T., R. Luukka, and G. Morton. 1978.
Journalism Quarterly 55(1).

Reading

Protocols for Environmental Reporting: What to Ask the Experts.
Fischhoff, B. 1985.
The Journalist. Winter, pp. 11-15.

Risk Communication: Facing Public Outrage.
Sandman, Peter M. 1987.
EPA Journal. November, pp. 21-22.

PAMPHLETS

Communicating Effectively About Risk Magnitudes.
Weinstein, Neil D., Peter M. Sandman, and Nancy E. Roberts. 1989.
New Brunswick, NJ: Environmental Communication Research Program, Rutgers University.

Explaining Environmental Risk.
Sandman, Peter M. 1986.
Washington, D.C.: U.S. Environmental Protection Agency.

Hazardous Substances in Our Environment: A Citizen's Guide to Understanding Health Risks and Reducing Exposure.
U.S. Environmental Protection Agency.
Washington D.C.: The Risk Communication Program, U. S. EPA. EPA-230-09-90-081.

Seven Cardinal Rules of Risk Communication.
U.S. Environmental Protection Agency. 1988.
Washington, D.C.: U. S. EPA. EPA-87-020.

Scientists and Journalists: Reporting Science as News.
Friedman, Sharon M., Sharon Dunwoody, and Carol L. Rogers. 1985.
Washington, D.C.: American Association for the Advancement of Science.

Index

Bold numbers indicate pages where key discussion of topic occurs.
Bold italic numbers indicate Glossary pages defining the term.

A

accumulation *99*
acute toxicity **30**, 32, 33, *99*
adsorption **23**
animal studies 5, 7, 9, 14, 28, **32**, 33, **35**, 37, **39**, 42, 68
association 44, **54**, 72, 77, *99*
average lethal dose **33**

B

bias 60, 61, **71**, 72–79, *99*
bioassay 31, 34, 38, **39**, 40, 41, 68, *99*
biologic credibility **54**

C

carcinogenesis bioassay 31, 34, 38, **39**, 40, 41, 68, *99*
case-control studies **48**, 50, 76, *100*
cases **48**, 73, 76
causation criteria **54**
chance 60, 61, **62**, 63–68, 70, 76
chemical properties **23**
chronic risks **94**
chronic toxicity **30**, 31, 34, *100*
classification errors **71**, 72, 73
clinical trials 51, **52**, *100*
clusters **55**, **56**, *100*
cohort studies 48, **49**, 50, 76, *100*
concentration analogies **93**, **98**
confidence intervals 62, **65**, **66**, 67, 68, *100*
confounders **77**, 78, 79, *100*
consistency **54**
controls, control groups **48**, 73, 76
cross-sectional studies **51**, *100*

D

dose-response concept **31**
dose-response studies 31, **35**, 36, 38, *101*
dose-response relationship **54**
double-blind **73**, *101*